MENINGITIS
100 MAXIMS

Volume 4 in the Series
100 Maxims in Neurology
Series Editor
Orrin Devinsky MD

OTHER VOLUMES IN THE SERIES

MENINGITIS
100 MAXIMS

Karen L Roos

Professor of Neurology,
Department of Neurology,
Indiana University School of Medicine,
Indianapolis, Indiana, USA

A member of the Hodder Headline Group
LONDON • SYDNEY • AUCKLAND
Co-published in the USA by
Oxford University Press, Inc., New York

First published in Great Britain 1996 by
Arnold, a member of the Hodder Headline Group
338 Euston Road, London NW1 3BH

Co-published in the United States by
Oxford University Press, Inc.,
198 Madison Avenue, New York, NY 10016
Oxford is a registered trademark of Oxford University Press

British Library Cataloguing in Publication Data
A catalogue record for this book is available from the British Library

Library of Congress Cataloging-in-Publication Data
A catalog record for this book is available from the Library of Congress

ISBN 0 340 60879 X

Typeset in 10/12 Palatino by
Textype Typesetters, Cambridge
Printed and bound in Great Britain by
J W Arrowsmith Ltd, Bristol

Contents

Chapter 1 History of Meningitis

Chapter 2 Pathogenesis and Pathophysiology of Bacterial Meningitis

Chapter 3 Clinical Presentation of Bacterial Meningitis

Chapter 4 Cerebrospinal Fluid (CSF)

Chapter 5 Etiologic Organism

Chapter 6 Therapy of Bacterial Meningitis

Chapter 7 Prevention of Bacterial Meningitis

Chapter 8 Aseptic Meningitis

Chapter 9 Fungal Meningitis

Chapter 10 Tuberculous Meningitis

Chapter 11 Syphilitic Meningitis

Chapter 12 Carcinomatous Meningitis

Foreword to the 100 Maxims in Neurology Series

The *100 Maxims in Neurology* series was originated by Roger Porter, MD. Based on his success with *Epilepsy: 100 Elementary Principles*, he recognized that this new approach in conceptualizing and presenting clinical information could extend well beyond epilepsy.

The basic principle of the *100 Maxims* is to bridge the gap between the didactic presentation of information in a review article or text with the clinical wisdom and pearls presented on clinical rounds or a phone consultation with a colleague. Experienced physicians make clinical decisions based on data from the literature, discussions with colleagues, and their own observations and lessons. The nuances of clinical neurology are thus often absent from the texts that provide careful and critical academic presentations.

Each maxim is intended to provide the reader with a clinical rule, a warning, an observation, or therapeutic principle. From the declarative statement, each maxim evolves as a brief clinical discussion, focusing on practical issues of pathophysiology, diagnosis or therapy. The goal is not a reference book, but a book that can be read from cover to cover and will confer a solid foundation of clinical knowledge. Selected references allow the interested reader to delve deeper into topics of interest.

As the baton of editorship passes from Roger Porter to me, the maxim series remains a new and poorly defined terrain in the ever expanding universe of neurology books. The maxim format holds great promise to teach neurology. Although the books are not "needed" by most neurologists – who will already have books in their libraries that cover the specific topics – the maxim books will provide an important tool for neurologists to practice their art. Standard textbooks summarize and present the "party line," often at the cost of avoiding controversy and making specific recommendations about the difficult clinical decisions. Idealized patients with black and white diagnoses exist mainly in textbooks. Doctors most often face gray zones and patients that fit into neither the square nor circular hole. The maxim texts are intended to address the gray zone where doctors practice medicine.

Creating and executing a new series of neurology books has been time consuming and challenging. My deepest thanks go to my family – Deborah, Janna and Julie – for providing the support and allowing the time.

Orrin Devinsky

Foreword to this Volume

Meningitis continues to claim many lives, despite the ability of antibiotics to destroy the deadly pathogens. It often emerges suddenly in a previously healthy child or adult but, if diagnosed and treated rapidly, neurologic outcome is excellent. A delay in diagnosis usually means morbidity or death. Meningitis stands as one of the few neurologic emergencies.

Dr Roos provides us with an informative and readable, thorough yet concise, overview of the major forms of meningitis – bacterial, viral, tuberculous, syphilitic, and carcinomatous. Covering pathophysiology, diagnosis and cerebrospinal fluid analysis, clinical features, and prevention and treatment, Dr Roos guides us through advances in our understanding and therapy, providing pearls and insights along the way.

This volume will prove invaluable to all physicians caring for children or adults. Meningitis can present in the office of the pediatrician, family physician, internist, or neurologist, in the emergency room, or in the hospital. It can strike at any age, with a predilection for the very young and very old. Meningitis can afflict those with no past medical history or patients with AIDS or cancer. Dr Roos's work helps us to understand and approach the many faces of this condition. Her maxims will prove helpful guides in clinical management. For example, there is comfort in the principle: "in the course of a lifetime, all conscientious physicians will have treated a number of cases of viral meningitis with a short course of antibiotics."

Dr Roos's *100 Maxims in Meningitis* fulfills the expectations of the best medical monograph – an expert has shared the wisdom of her clinical and research experience and thorough knowledge of the literature. This book should be warmly welcomed by all residents and attending physicians.

Orin Devinsky MD
1996

Preface

Meningitis is a devastating neurologic disease of infancy, childhood and adulthood. Despite effective antimicrobial therapy, the morbidity and mortality from this infection remain high. Over the last 10 years our increasing understanding of the pathophysiology of the neurologic complications of meningitis has turned our attention not only to treating the infection, but also to anticipating and treating the neurologic complications with the hope of eventually preventing them. Despite effective antimicrobial therapy, the care of these patients continues to be difficult, as coma, seizure activity and stroke complicate the course of the disease. Fungal, tuberculous and syphilitic meningitis are increasing in incidence with the increasing numbers of immunocompromised patients. Although the recognition of carcinomatous meningitis is fairly straightforward, the treatment of this form of meningitis is primarily aimed at prolonging survival. This book was written for the clinician as an aid in the care of patients, and for resident doctors and students to gain an understanding of this disease. It is my hope in this Decade of the Brain and beyond that we will continue to gain an increasing understanding of the pathophysiology of neurologic complications of central nervous system infections so that we can not only improve survival but also improve the neurologic outcome.

Karen L Roos MD

Acknowledgements

I would like to acknowledge and thank our administrative supervisor, Linda Hagan, for her technical support. I also want to thank Kenneth E Greer, Chairman of Dermatology at the University of Virginia, for providing figures of skin lesions, and Sharon Teal for medical illustration. I wish to extend my heart-felt thanks to my husband, Robert M Pascuzzi, MD, who helped in the care of my patients, our students and resident doctors, and our children so that this manuscript could be written. This book is dedicated to him and to our daughters, Annie and Jan.

1
History of Meningitis

1. Meningitis was first accurately described around 1800

Robert Whytt initially described symptoms and signs of tuberculous meningitis in 1768 and called this "dropsy in the brain". He considered the collection of fluid in the ventricles as the disease itself, most likely because at the end of the eighteenth century the ventricles were regarded as the seat of the soul. Physicians at that time attributed somnolence and coma to a collection of fluid in the "seat of the soul" (i.e. "acute hydrocephalus"). By the end of the eighteenth century, investigators were beginning to shift their attention from the ventricles to the meninges.[1]

Meningococcal meningitis, or as it was previously called, "cerebrospinal fever", was first described by Gaspard Vieusseux on a small outbreak in Geneva in 1805.[2]

The first epidemic of spotted fever to be documented in America was in Medfield, Massachusetts, in 1806 and is recorded in the Medical and Agricultural Register for the years 1806–7.[3] Nine people died. Drs Elias Mann and Lothario Danielson describe the clinical presentation as follows:

> Without any apparent predisposition, the patient is suddenly taken with violent pain in the head and stomach, succeeded by cold chills and followed by nausea and puking; and in a child of 15 months old, a very violent pulsation was discovered at the fontanel . . . the eyes have a wild vacant stare; these symptoms are accompanied by a peculiar fearfulness, as if in danger of falling from the bed or nurse's arms, and continue from six to nine hours, when coma (suppression of sense and voluntary motion) commences, with increasing debility; extremities become cold; livid spots resembling petechiae (purple spots which appear in the last stages of certain fevers) appear under the skin, on the face, neck, and extremities; spasms occur at intervals, which increase in violence and frequency in proportion as the force of the circulation decreases; at this time the eyes appear glassy, and the size of the pupil varies suddenly, from almost wholly obliterating the iris, down to the size of a millet seed, and then again as suddenly dilating. These symptoms seem to mark the second period of the disease, and continue from three to five hours. The third and last stage is distinguished by a total loss of pulsation at the wrists; livid appearances become more general; spasms more violent; coma more profound; death!
>
> The report of autopsy examination reads as follows:
> On removing the cranium, and dividing the dura mater, there was

discharged, by estimation half an ounce of serus fluid. The dura and pia mater in several places adhered together and both to the substance of the brain. The veins of the brain were uncommonly turgid with a fluid similar to that which was discharged from between its membranes, and the substance of the brain itself remarkably soft, offering scarcely any resistance to the finger when thrust into it.[3]

Several different treatment modalities were employed. Initially, much emphasis was placed on evacuating the stomach and bowels. The treatment of meningitis in 1806 consisted of repeated stomach and bowel evacuations, inducing sweating by placing blocks of hemlock boiled in water and wrapped in cloth next to the patient and "the stimulating powers of bark and wine".[3,4]

The recognition of meningismus as a diagnostic sign of meningitis is credited to a medical student, Nathan Strong. As a requirement for his medical degree he presented an "Inaugural Dissertation on the Disease Termed Petechial or Spotted Fever" to the Medical Society of Connecticut in 1810. In his dissertation the following description appears: "the extensor muscles of the head and neck were, in almost every case, affected with tonic spasm". Vladimir Mihailovich Kernig described his maneuver for detecting meningeal irritation in 1882, and Jozef Brudzinski described at least five different meningeal signs in 1909 recognizing that some may be present while others are absent.[5]

The first patient on whom Heinrich Quincke performed a lumbar puncture reportedly had meningococcal meningitis, and Quincke is credited with describing the technique of lumbar puncture (1891)[6], though Heubner was the first to recover "biscuit-shaped" meningococci from the spinal fluid.[7,8] Anton Weichselbaum is credited with identifying the meningococcus in 1887, and describing it as the *Diplococcus intracellularis meningitidis*.[9]

References

1. Mullener ER. Six Geneva physicians on meningitis. *J Hist Med* 1965; **20**: 1–3.
2. Vieusseux G. Memoire sur la maladie qui a regne a Geneve au printemps de 1805. *J Med Chi Pharm* 1806; **11**: 163–82.
3. Danielson L, Mann E. The history of a singular and very mortal disease which lately made its appearance in Medfield. In: Adams B (ed.), *The Medical and Agricultural Register*. Boston, MA: Manning and Loring, 1806, p. 65–9.
4. Grady FJ. Some early American reports on meningitis: with special reference to the Inaugural Dissertation of Nathan Strong. *J Hist Med* 1965; **20**: 27–32.
5. Verghese A, Gallemore G. Kernig's and Brudzinski's signs revisited. *Rev Infect Dis* 1987; **9**: 1187–92.
6. Quincke H. *Uber hydrocephalus, Verhandlungen des Congressus fur innere Medizin, Vol 10*. Wiesbaden: JF Bergman, 1891, 321.
7. Blackfan KD. The treatment of meningococcus meningitis. *Medicine* 1922; **1**: 139–212.
8. Heubner O. Beobachtungen und Versuche uber den Meningococcus intracellularis

(Weichselbaum-Jaeger). *Jahrb Kinderheilk* 1896; **43**: 1.
9. Weichselbaum A. Über die Ätiologie der Akuten Meningitis cerebro-spinalis. *Fortschr Med* 1887; **5**: 573.

2.   *The history of the treatment of meningitis is the history of antibacterial therapy*

In the late nineteenth century, meningitis was treated by drainage of CSF by repeated lumbar punctures. At the turn of the century, Jochmann in Germany and Flexner in New York began experiments that demonstrated the protective effect of antimeningococcal serum in experimental meningococcal infections in animals.[1,2] The subcutaneous and intravenous administration of antisera therapy initially proved disappointing in treating this infection in humans and Flexner proposed the antisera be administered by intraspinal injection. In 1913, Flexner reported the results of 1294 cases of meningococcal meningitis that had been treated with intrathecal injections of "antimeningitis serum". Anti-serum (20–30 mL) was administered by intrathecal injection after 30–40 mL of CSF had been withdrawn and was continued daily for 4 days. Persistent or worsening symptoms were treated with additional injections. The survival rate increased from between 10% and 30% in untreated patients to 69.1% in 1294 cases treated with antimeningococcal serum.[3,4]

The discovery of the antibacterial activity of sulfonamides in the early 1930s ushered in the antibiotic era. The successful treatment of President Franklin Roosevelt's son for a streptococcal throat infection with a sulfonamide was reported in the *New York Times* in 1936 and was probably significant in making sulfonamides widely available to American physicians soon thereafter.[3]

Francis Schwentker is credited with the first demonstration of a cure of meningococcal meningitis with sulfanilamide therapy. Schwentker et al.[5] reported the survival of nine patients with meningococcal meningitis. Sulfanilamide solution (10–30 mL) was injected intraspinally into the patient after a slightly larger volume of spinal fluid had been removed. A larger amount of the solution was given subcutaneously. Both the intraspinal and subcutaneous treatments were repeated every 12 hours for the first 2 days and once each day thereafter until definite improvement was evident. Ten cases of meningococcal meningitis were treated and only one patient died, and that was from pneumonia. Sulfonamide therapy so improved survival from meningococcal meningitis that it was called a "miracle drug" and the effect of these agents in desperately ill patients was likened to "divine intervention".[6]

In the early part of the twentieth century, the other two major pathogens that cause meningitis today, *Streptococcus pneumoniae* and *Haemophilus influenzae*, had not caused epidemics comparable to those seen with *Neisseria meningitidis*.[7] *Mycobacterium tuberculosis* and *N. meningitidis* were the two most common causative organisms of meningitis. Prior to the antibiotic era, the treatment of meningitis caused by *S. pneumoniae* and *H. influenzae* was similar to that of meningococcal meningitis with drainage of CSF and antiserum therapy. The prognosis of meningitis caused by these organisms was grave. Of 99 patients with pneumococcal meningitis hospitalized in the Boston City Hospital between 1920 and 1936, the mortality rate was 100%.[7,8] In 1937, the mortality rate from *H. influenzae* meningitis in children was 98%.[9] By the end of the 1930s, the mortality rate for *H. influenzae* meningitis had decreased to 25% due to sulfonamide therapy.[10] Flemming discovered penicillin in 1931. Between the years 1950 and 1961 bacterial meningitis of unknown etiology was treated as follows: sulfadiazine for meningococcus, penicillin for pneumococcus and chloramphenicol for *H. influenzae*.[3] The identification of sulfadiazine-resistant meningococcal organisms brought an end to the sulfonamide era of therapy for meningitis.[3]

The Second World War brought an epidemic of meningococcal meningitis in US servicemen. From 1940 to 1945, 14,504 hospital admissions of military personnel were due to this disease.[11]

In 1944 Rosenberg and Arling[12] reported their success in treating 65 patients with cerebrospinal fever (in 50 cases meningococci grew in culture and 15 cases were diagnosed on clinical presentation). In most cases penicillin was given intravenously for the first 8 hours and continued intramuscularly (10,000 units) every 3 hours thereafter. Penicillin (10,000 units) was administered intrathecally at 24-hour intervals until clinical improvement, a decrease in temperature and/or a decrease in meningeal signs was evident, and until the stained smears and cultures of the spinal fluid revealed no organisms. In the most severe infections and in those in which the patient was comatose, intrathecal penicillin was continued until the spinal fluid was free of bacteria on three successive days. The authors discuss not only the importance of draining CSF before injecting penicillin but the difficulties encountered in draining "viscous" CSF. Rosenberg and Arling used comparatively low doses of systemic penicillin in their patients. It was not until around 1950 that the first clinical trials using high doses of systemic penicillin alone were reported and the intrathecal instillation of penicillin was no longer required for therapeutic success.[7]

References

1. Jochmann G. Versuche zur Serodiagnostik und Serotherapie der epidemischen Genickstarre. *Deutsche med Wehnschr* 1906; **32**: 788.
2. Flexner S. Experimental cerebrospinal meningitis and its serum treatment. *JAMA* 1906; **47**: 560.
3. Scheld WM, Mandell GL. Sulfonamides and meningitis. *JAMA* 1984; **251**: 791–4.
4. Flexner S. The results of the serum treatment in thirteen hundred cases of epidemic meningitis. *J Exp Med* 1913; **17**: 553–76.

5. Schwentker FF, Gelman S, Long PH. The treatment of meningococcic meningitis with sulfanilamide. *JAMA* 1984; **251:** 788–90.
6. McDermott W, Rogers DE. Social ramifications of control of microbial disease. *Johns Hopkins Med J* 1982; **151:** 302–12.
7. Tauber MG, Sande MA. The impact of penicillin on the treatment of meningitis. *JAMA* 1984; **251:** 1877–80.
8. Finland M, Brown JW, Rauh AE. Treatment of pneumococci meningitis. *N Engl J Med* 1938; **218:** 1033–44.
9. Fothergill LD. *Hemophilus influenzae* (Pfeiffer bacillus) meningitis and its specific treatment. *N Engl J Med* 1937; **216:** 587–90.
10. Alexander HE. Treatment of type b *Haemophilus influenzae* meningitis. *J Pediatr* 1944; **25:** 517–32.
11. Bell WE, Silber DL. Meningococcal meningitis: past and present concepts. *Military Medicine* 1971; **136:** 601–11.
12. Rosenberg DH, Arling PA. Penicillin in the treatment of meningitis. *JAMA* 1944; **125:** 1011–17.

2

Pathogenesis and Pathophysiology of Bacterial Meningitis

3. Meningeal pathogens initially colonize the nasopharynx

The most common bacteria that cause meningitis, *Haemophilus influenzae*, *Neisseria meningitidis* and *Streptococcus pneumoniae* initially colonize the nasopharynx by attaching to the nasopharyngeal epithelial cells. In order to attach to the mucosal epithelial cells, *H. influenzae*, *N. meningitidis* and *S. pneumoniae* secrete IgA proteases that break down the mucous barrier allowing bacterial attachment to the epithelium. The organism then attaches to the nasopharyngeal epithelial cells via an interaction between bacterial surface structures, such as finger-like projections (pili) and host cell surface receptors. After the bacteria have successfully attached to the nasopharyngeal epithelial cells, they are either carried across the cell in membrane-bound vacuoles to the intravascular space or, as in the case of *H. influenzae*, create separations in the apical tight junctions of columnar epithelial cells and invade primarily by an intercellular route.[1]

Once the bacteria gain access to the bloodstream, they are successful in avoiding phagocytosis by neutrophils because of the presence of a polysaccharide capsule. In addition, the polysaccharide capsule allows the organism to evade the complement pathway – the chief initial host defense against bacteremia. Bacteria that are able to survive in the circulation then enter the CSF through the choroid plexus of the lateral ventricles, and other areas of altered blood–brain barrier permeability. Cells in the choroid plexus and cerebral capillaries possess receptors for adherence of specific bacterial cell-surface structures that allow for attachment and adherence of meningeal pathogens.[2,3]

Once meningeal pathogens gain access to the CSF, there are insufficient complement components, immunoglobulin concentrations and neutrophils in the subarachnoid space to retard their rapid multiplication. The CSF is an area of impaired host defense. Normal uninfected CSF contains no phagocytic cells, has a low protein concentration, contains no IgM, and has low levels of C_3 and C_4.[4] The opsonization of bacteria by complement and immunoglobulins is an essential step for phagocytosis by neutrophils; however, opsonic activity is virtually undetectable in the CSF of normal subjects, and is insufficient in the CSF of patients with meningitis for bacterial lysis or opsonization.[4,5] Like complement, immunoglobulin concentrations are low in the CSF of uninfected individuals, and increase only slightly in the course of bacterial meningitis. This typically occurs late in the disease process. As a result of the lack of opsonization of bacteria by complement and immunoglobulins, the phagocytosis of bacteria by leukocytes is inefficient and consequently the multiplication of bacteria in the subarachnoid space rapidly overcomes the clearance mechanisms of the CSF.

References

1. Quagliarello V, Scheld WM. Bacterial meningitis: pathogenesis, pathophysiology, and progress. *N Engl J Med* 1992; **327**: 864–72.
2. Parkkinen J, Korhonen T, Pere A, Hacker J, Soinila S. Binding sites in the rat brain for *Escherichia coli* S fimbriae associated with neonatal meningitis. *J Clin Invest* 1988; **81**: 860–5.
3. Roos KL, Tunkel AR, Scheld WM. Acute bacterial meningitis in children and adults. In: Scheld WM, Whitley RJ, Durack DT (eds), *Infections of the Central Nervous System*. New York: Raven Press, 1991; 335–410.
4. Zwahlen A, Nydegger UE, Vaudaux P, Lambert PH, Waldvogel FA. Complement-mediated opsonic activity in normal and infected human cerebrospinal fluid: early response during bacterial meningitis. *J Infect Dis* 1982; **145**: 635–46.
5. Simberkoff MS, Moldover NH, Rahal J Jr. Absence of detectable bactericidal and opsonic activities in normal and infected human cerebrospinal fluids: a regional host defense deficiency. *J Lab Clin Med* 1980; **95**: 362–72.

4. *The release of bacterial cell-wall components by the lysis of bacteria in the subarachnoid space is the initial step in the induction of meningeal inflammation*

In William Osler's description of "cerebro-spinal fever" in 1912 the following account appears:

> The exudate is usually fibrino-purulent, most marked at the base of the brain, where the meninges may be greatly thickened and plastered over with it. Sometimes the entire cortex is covered with a thick, purulent exudate.
> Danielson and Mann made five autopsies and were the first to describe "a fluid resembling pus between the dura and pia mater".[1]

The mechanism by which meningeal inflammation develops is now understood. It is not simply the presence of bacteria in the subarachnoid space that induces the inflammatory response, but rather the presence of bacterial cell-wall components due to lysis of bacteria that induces the inflammatory response. The lipo-oligosaccharide (LOS) component of the

Haemophilus influenzae type b (Hib) cell wall, and cell-wall components of the pneumococcus, specifically lipoteichoic acid, have been demonstrated in experimental models of meningitis to induce meningeal inflammation. These are encapsulated pathogens, but the capsular polysaccharide does not appear to contribute to the ability of these organisms to produce meningeal inflammation.[2,3] Gram-negative bacteria have lipopolysaccharide (LPS) molecules (endotoxin) attached to their outer membranes. The endotoxin of *H. influenzae* has a shorter saccharide chain, thus the designation LOS.

Syrogiannopoulos et al.[2] investigated the ability of Hib LOS to induce meningeal inflammation in rabbits. The intracisternal inoculation of 2 fg–200 ng of LOS produced a dose-dependent increase in the concentration of white blood cells and protein in CSF and the development of a meningeal exudate. The lipid A region of Hib LOS appears to be responsible for eliciting the inflammatory response based on the following observations in experimental models of meningitis:

1. polymyxin B, an antibiotic that is able to neutralize the bioactivities of LPS by binding to the lipid A region of the molecule, is able to significantly reduce the inflammatory potency of Hib LOS;
2. neutrophil acyloxyacyl hydrolase, an enzyme that is able to remove nonhydroxylated fatty acids from the lipid A region of LOS, also reduces the tissue toxicity of LOS.[2]

The LPS molecule, or endotoxin, also appears to play a significant role in the alteration of the blood–brain barrier permeability. Wispelwey et al.[4] observed that the intracisternal inoculation of Hib LPS into rats resulted in a profound increase in blood–brain barrier permeability. This alteration in blood–brain barrier permeability is significant in its contribution to vasogenic brain edema. The profound effects that Hib LPS exerts on blood–brain barrier permeability in meningeal inflammation raises questions about our current antibiotic treatment of bacterial meningitis. It appears that it is the free LPS and not the cell-associated LPS that is responsible for the observed effects of this molecule. Bactericidal antibiotics that lead to the release of free LPS may be, at least transiently, detrimental to the host.[4] Similarly, fragments of the pneumococcal cell wall can induce inflammation in the CSF.[3] Antibiotics that kill gram-negative bacteria by cell wall lysis with the subsequent release of endotoxin have been shown in experimental models of meningitis to be associated with a dramatic increase in vasogenic brain edema.[5]

The effect of antimicrobial therapy on CSF endotoxin levels was measured in children with *H. influenzae* meningitis. There was a significant increase in levels of free endotoxin in CSF after the institution of therapy with bacteriolytic antibiotics. This increase in CSF free endotoxin was accompanied by a significant increase in the levels of CSF lactate and LDH of white blood cell origin (due to increased inflammation), and a decrease in the level of CSF glucose suggesting a shift to anaerobic glycolysis by the brain. This observation of an increase in the free endotoxin level in CSF after the initiation of therapy in children with bacterial meningitis may contribute to our understanding of the etiology of cerebrovascular disease in this infection. In a primate model of *H. influenzae* meningitis, a reduction in cerebrocortical blood flow was observed to correlate with cisternal CSF LPS concentrations. The intracisternal injection of *Escherichia coli* LPS in the primate model produced a marked decline in total cerebrocortical blood flow.[6,7] A significant association has also been observed between CSF LPS concentrations of >1000 ng/ml and the development of seizures.[7] A direct relationship between the concentration of CSF endotoxin and outcome of neonatal gram-negative meningitis has been reported.[8] In addition there is a strong correlation between CSF LPS concentrations and the development of seizures, and morbidity and mortality in children with gram-negative meningitis.[7-9]

References

1. Osler W, McCrae T. Cerebro-spinal fever. In: *Principles and Practice of Medicine*. New York: D. Appleton & Company, 1912; 108–15.
2. Syrogiannopoulos GA, Hansen EJ, Erwin AL, Munford RS, Rutledge J, Reisch JS, McCracken GH. *Haemophilus influenzae* type b lipooligosaccharide induces meningeal inflammation. *J Infect Dis* 1988; **157**: 237–44.
3. Tuomanen E, Tomasz A, Hengstler B, Zak O. The relative role of bacterial cell wall and capsule in the induction of inflammation in pneumococcal meningitis. *J Infect Dis* 1985; **151**: 535–40.
4. Wispelwey B, Lesse AJ, Hansen EJ, Scheld WM. *Haemophilus influenzae* lipopolysaccharide-induced blood brain barrier permeability during experimental meningitis in the rat. *J Clin Invest* 1988; **82**: 1339–46.
5. Tauber MG, Shibl AM, Hackbarth CJ, Larrick JW, Sande MA. Antibiotic therapy, endotoxin concentration in cerebrospinal fluid, and brain edema in experimental *Escherichia coli* meningitis in the rat. *J Infect Dis* 1987; **156**: 456–61.
6. Smith AL, Scheifele D, Daun R, Averill D, Syriopolou V. Cerebral blood flow in experimental *Haemophilus influenzae* b meningitis. *Pediatr Infect Dis J* 1987; 6(suppl): 1159.
7. Arditi M, Ables L, Yogev R. Cerebrospinal fluid endotoxin levels in children with *H. influenzae* meningitis before and after administration of intravenous ceftriaxone. *J Infect Dis* 1989; **160**: 1005–11.
8. McCracken GH Jr, Sarff LD. Endotoxin in cerebrospinal fluid: detection in neonates with bacterial meningitis. *JAMA* 1976; **235**: 617–20.
9. Dwelle TL, Dunkle LM, Blair L. Correlation of cerebrospinal fluid endotoxin activity with clinical and laboratory variables in gram-negative bacterial meningitis in children. *J Clin Microbiol* 1987; **25**: 856–8.

5.   Bacterial cell-wall components stimulate the production of the inflammatory cytokines, interleukin-1 and tumor necrosis factor, which subsequently induce meningeal inflammation

In experimental models of meningitis, within 1–3 hours after the intracisternal inoculation of lipopolysaccharide, tumor necrosis factor (TNF) and interleukin-1 (IL-1) activity are present in CSF followed by the onset of the inflammatory process (increased concentrations of protein and leukocytes in CSF). Both IL-1 and TNF are produced by monocytes, macrophages, and brain astrocytes and microglial cells (CNS macrophage-equivalent cells). The synthesis and release of IL-1 and TNF are stimulated by lipopolysaccharide (LPS), by lipoteichoic acid and by each other.[1–5]

As can be seen from Fig. 5.1, the induction of an inflammatory response in the subarachnoid space is the critical event leading to the neurologic complications of bacterial meningitis. The biological activities of TNF relevant to its role as an inflammatory mediator in bacterial meningitis include:

1. promotion of neutrophil adherence to vascular endothelial cells;
2. induction of IL-1 synthesis and release from activated astrocytes and microglial cells.

One of the major contributors to the purulent exudate in the subarachnoid space during meningitis is a CSF neutrophilic pleocytosis. The precise mechanism by which neutrophils traverse the blood–brain barrier is unknown. However, it appears that the adherence of neutrophils to vascular endothelial cells is a necessary prerequisite. Specific adhesion molecules are required on vascular endothelial cells for the adhesion of neutrophils. The inflammatory cytokines, IL-1 and TNF, induce the formation of endothelial leukocyte adhesion molecules. These receptors are necessary for the movement of leukocytes across the blood–brain barrier.[6] In experimental meningitis, TNF activity is first detected in the CSF of rabbits 45 minutes after intracisternal inoculation of *Haemophilus influenzae* type b (Hib) lipo-oligosaccharide (LOS) and persists for approximately 5 hours. A similar response is seen in human subjects given endotoxin intravenously. The presence of a CSF pleocytosis is observed 75 minutes after TNF is detected.[7] The presence of neutrophils in the subarachnoid space is both detrimental and beneficial to the host. It is not clear what role, if any, neutrophils play in eradicating the infection in the subarachnoid space. In experimental studies of pneumococcal meningitis, there is no significant difference in the bacterial growth rate in CSF in animals that are leukopenic compared with controls.[8]

The presence of TNF in CSF appears to be specific for bacterial meningitis. Elevated concentrations of TNF were observed in 42 of 51 patients (82%) with purulent bacterial meningitis, and in only 5 of 78 individuals with nonbacterial meningitis. The individuals with nonbacterial meningitis and elevated concentrations of TNF in CSF had either herpes simplex type 2 or

PATHOPHYSIOLOGY OF BACTERIAL MENINGITIS

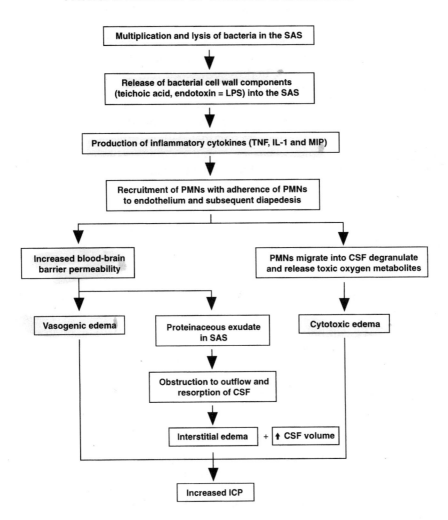

SAS = Subarachnoid Space, LPS = Lipopolysaccharide, TNF = Tumor Necrosis Factor ∝,
IL-1 = Interleukin-1, MIP = Macrophage Inflammatory Protein, ICP = Intracranial Pressure

Fig. 5.1   The neurologic complications of bacterial meningitis are the result of an inflammatory cascade of events that is initiated by the multiplication and lysis of bacteria in the subarachnoid space.

varicella-zoster virus meningitis.[9] These observations have been supported by the results of other clinical studies. Arditi et al.[10] detected TNF activity in the CSF of 33 of 38 children with bacterial meningitis. TNF was undetectable in the CSF of 15 children with viral meningitis/encephalitis.[10] Tumor necrosis factor activity was detected in the initial CSF samples from 90% of neonates with gram-negative meningitis, but in none of 34 children with aseptic meningitis.[11,12] Arditi et al.[10] also found a significant association between admission CSF TNF concentrations greater than 1000 pg/mL and the development of seizures, and hypothesized that CSF TNF activity may contribute to seizure activity through local metabolic and vascular effects. Waage et al.[13] found a strong correlation between admission serum TNF levels and mortality in patients with meningococcal meningitis; patients with serum TNF concentrations greater than 140 pg/mL died.

Tumor necrosis factor also has a role in the induction of the synthesis and release of IL-1. Interleukin-1 has the following biological activities:

1. chemoattractant for neutrophils;
2. the induction of proliferative responses in many tissues, including the brain, where IL-1-induced proliferation of glial cells may contribute to brain gliosis (scarring);
3. the stimulation of neutrophils to degranulate and release toxic oxygen metabolites that then increase blood–brain barrier permeability.[3]

When human recombinant IL-1 was inoculated intracisternally into adult rats, there was a dose-dependent increase in the degree of meningeal inflammation. Pre-incubation of human recombinant IL-1 with a monoclonal antibody against it significantly inhibited the inflammatory response, providing good evidence of the role of IL-1 in inducing meningeal inflammation.[7,14]

Interleukin-1 may have a role in the altered level of consciousness and the production of fever in bacterial meningitis. It has been demonstrated that IL-1 facilitates slow-wave sleep and produces fever by its effect on the hypothalamus.[15,16] Mustafa et al.[17] demonstrated detectable concentrations of IL-1 beta at the time of diagnosis in 95% of aliquots of CSF from 102 infants and children with bacterial meningitis. The infants and children with initial CSF IL-1 beta concentrations greater than or equal to 500 pg per ml were more likely to have neurologic sequelae than the infants and children with lower CSF IL-1 beta concentrations. In addition, the CSF IL-1 beta concentration correlated directly with CSF leukocyte count, lactate, protein and tumor necrosis factor concentrations, and inversely with the CSF glucose concentration.

Other inflammatory cytokines have a role in the induction of meningeal inflammation. Tumor necrosis factor alpha and IL-1 are potent inducers of the synthesis and release of platelet-activating factor (PAF) from various cells including polymorphonuclear leukocytes, macrophages/monocytes, endothelial cells and neuronal cells. Platelet-activating factor has the following biological activities:

1. the recruitment and activation of neutrophils and monocytes to the site of inflammation;
2. a direct toxicity to neuronal cells;
3. synergistic activity with lipopolysaccharide and TNF-alpha in the development of microvascular tissue damage;
4. the induction of structural changes of vascular endothelial cells leading to increased capillary permeability and edema formation.[10]

Other inflammatory cytokines, such as interleukin-6, have also been detected in the CSF of patients with bacterial meningitis.

The arachidonic acid metabolites, prostaglandins E_2 and I_2 have been detected in the CSF of infants and children with bacterial meningitis.[18] Prostaglandin E_2 has been detected in the CSF of rabbits with pneumococcal meningitis.[19-21] In addition, IL-1 beta and TNF stimulate phospholipase A_2 activity, the enzyme which releases arachidonic acids from membrane phospholipids. Prostaglandins are important mediators of systemic inflammatory processes, although their exact contribution to the pathophysiology of bacterial meningitis is unknown.

References

1. Townsend GC, Scheld WM. Adjunctive therapy for bacterial meningitis: rationale for use, current status, and prospects for the future. *Clin Infect Dis* 1993; **17**(Suppl 2): S537–49.
2. Beutler B, Mahoney J, Le Trang N, Pekala P, Cerami A. Purification of cachectin, a lipoprotein lipase-suppressing hormone secreted by endotoxin-induced RAW 264.7 cells. *J Exp Med* 1985; **161**: 984–95.
3. Dinarello CA. Interleukin-1. *Rev Infect Dis* 1984; **6**: 51–95.
4. Bhakdi S, Klonish T, Nuber P, Fischer W. Stimulation of monokine production by lipoteichoic acids. *Infect Immun* 1991; **59**: 4614–20.
5. Le J, Vilcek J. Tumor necrosis factor and interleukin 1: cytokines with multiple overlapping biological activities. *Lab Invest* 1987; **56**: 234–48.
6. Tunkel AR, Wispelwey B, Scheld WM. Bacterial meningitis: recent advances in pathophysiology and treatment. *Ann Intern Med* 1990; **112**: 610–23.
7. Saez-Llorens X, Ramilo O, Mustafa MM, Mertsola J, McCracken GH. Molecular pathophysiology of bacterial meningitis: current concepts and therapeutic implications. *J Pediatr* 1990; **116**: 671–84.
8. Ernst JD, Decazes JM, Sande MA. Experimental pneumococcal meningitis: role of leukocytes in pathogenesis. *Infect Immun* 1983; **41**: 275–9.
9. Glimaker M, Kragsbjerg P, Forsgren M, Olcen P. Tumor necrosis factor-alpha (TNF-alpha) in cerebrospinal fluid from patients with meningitis of different etiologies: high levels of TNF-alpha indicate bacterial meningitis. *J Infect Dis* 1993; **167**: 882–9.
10. Arditi M, Manogue KR, Caplan M, Yogev R. Cerebrospinal fluid cachectin/tumor necrosis factor-alpha and platelet-activating factor concentrations and severity of bacterial meningitis in children. *J Infect Dis* 1990; **162**: 139–47.
11. McCracken GH Jr, Mustafa MM, Ramilo O, Olsen KD, Risser RC. Cerebrospinal fluid interleukin 1-beta and tumor necrosis factor concentrations and outcome

from neonatal gram-negative enteric bacillary meningitis. *Pediatr Infect Dis J* 1989; **8**: 155–9.

12. Ramilo O, Mustafa MM, Porter J, Olsen KD, Luby J, McCracken GH Jr. Concentrations of IL-1 beta and TNF in CSF of infants and children with meningitis (abstract 1108). *Pediatr Res* 1989; **25**(Part 2): 187A.

13. Waage A, Halstensen A, Espevik T. Association between tumour necrosis factor in serum and fatal outcome in patients with meningococcal disease. *Lancet* 1987; **i**: 355–7.

14. Scheld WM, Quagliarello VJ, Wispelwey B. The potential role of host cytokines in *Haemophilus influenzae* lipopolysaccharide-induced blood–brain barrier permeability. *Pediatr Infect Dis J* 1989; **8**: 910–11.

15. Dinarello CA. An update on human interleukin-1: from molecular biology to clinical relevance. *J Clin Immunol* 1985; **5**: 287–96.

16. Kruger J, Dinarello C, Chedid L. Promotion of slow wave sleep by a purified interleukin-1 preparation. *Fed Proc* 1983; **42**: 356.

17. Mustafa MM, Lebel MH, Ramilo O, Olsen KD, et al. Correlation of interleukin-1 beta and cachectin concentrations in cerebrospinal fluid and outcome from bacterial meningitis. *J Pediatr* 1989; **115**: 208–13.

18. Mustafa MM, Ramilo O, Saez-Llorens X, Olsen KD, et al. Cerebrospinal fluid prostaglandins, Interleukin-1 beta, and tumor necrosis factor in bacterial meningitis. *Am J Dis Child* 1990; **144**: 883–7.

19. Tureen JH, Stella FB, Clyman RI, Mauroy F, Sande MA. Effect of indomethacin on brain water content, cerebrospinal fluid white blood cell response and prostaglandin E_2 levels in cerebrospinal fluid in experimental meningitis in rabbits. *Pediatr Infect Dis J* 1987; **6**: 1151–3.

20. Kadurugamuwa JL, Hengstler B, Zak O. Effects of anti-inflammatory drugs on arachidonic acid metabolites and cerebrospinal fluid proteins during infectious pneumococcal meningitis in rabbits. *Pediatr Infect Dis J* 1987; **6**: 1153–4.

21. Tuomanen E, Hengstler B, Rich R, Bray MA, Zak O, Tomasz A. Nonsteroidal antiinflammatory agents in the therapy for experimental pneumococcal meningitis. *J Infect Dis* 1987; **155**: 985–90.

6. The alteration in blood–brain barrier permeability during bacterial meningitis results in vasogenic cerebral edema and increased intracranial pressure, and allows for the leakage of plasma proteins into the CSF

The major sites of the blood–brain barrier are the arachnoid membrane, the choroid plexus epithelium and the endothelial cells of the cerebral blood vessels. The cerebral capillary endothelium is able to function as a high-resistance endothelium and serve as a barrier to circulating macromolecules, such as albumin, because of unique ultrastructural properties that distinguish cerebral capillaries from systemic capillaries. Cerebral capillary endothelial cells are fused together by tight junctions (zonulae occludens) that prevent intercellular transport, and pinocytotic vesicles are rare or absent in cerebral capillary endothelial cells.

In early studies of the mechanism of infection-induced breakdown of the blood–brain barrier in rats, isolated cerebral microvessels were examined ultrastructurally after the experimental induction of meningitis. There was an increase in cytoplasmic pinocytotic vesicles and complete separation of the intercellular tight junctions in the microvessels. The morphologic alterations in cerebral microvessels were identical during meningitis induced by different types of encapsulated bacteria (*Haemophilus influenzae*, *Streptococcus pneumoniae*, and *Escherichia coli*) and correlated with the exit of ^{125}I-labeled albumin into the CSF.[1]

Bacterial meningitis increases the permeability of the blood–brain barrier at the level of the choroid plexus epithelium and the endothelial cells of the cerebral microvasculature.[2] The inflammatory cytokines, interleukin-1 (IL-1) and tumor necrosis factor (TNF), act synergistically in altering the permeability of the blood–brain barrier. In experimental meningitis models, this effect on the cerebral capillary endothelium by IL-1 and TNF has been demonstrated by an increase in the penetration of ^{125}I-labeled albumin from serum into CSF.[3,4] The major pathophysiologic consequence of an increased blood–brain barrier permeability is vasogenic edema and the exudation of serum proteins into the CSF. The presence of leukocytes in CSF appears to enhance blood–brain barrier permeability late in the disease course. Vasogenic edema contributes to the development of increased intracranial pressure. Significant increases in intracranial pressure are associated not only with a risk of cerebral herniation but also a decrease in cerebral perfusion pressure. The adherence of leukocytes to capillary endothelial cells increases the permeability of blood vessels, allowing the leakage of plasma proteins into the CSF and contributing to the inflammatory exudate in the subarachnoid space.

References

1. Quagliarello V, Scheld WM. Bacterial meningitis: pathogenesis,pathophysiology, and progress. *New Engl J Med* 1992; **327:** 864–72.
2. Tunkel AR, Wispelwey B, Scheld WM. Bacterial meningitis: recent advances in pathophysiology and treatment. *Ann Intern Med* 1990; **112:** 610–23.
3. Mustafa MM, Lebel MH, Ramilo O, Olsen KD, et al. Correlation of interleukin-1 beta and cachectin concentrations in cerebrospinal fluid and outcome from bacterial meningitis. *J Pediatr* 1989; **115:** 208–13.
4. Wispelwey B, Long JM, Castracane JM, Scheld WM. Cerebrospinal fluid interleukin-1 activity following intracisternal inoculation of *Haemophilus influenzae* lipooligosaccharide. Presented to the 28th Interscience Conference on Antimicrobial Agents and Chemotherapy, Los Angeles, California, October 26, 1988.

7.   Increased intracranial pressure in bacterial meningitis is due to a combination of cerebral edema, an increased volume of CSF, and an increase in cerebral blood volume

The cerebral edema that develops in the course of bacterial meningitis is due to a combination of vasogenic, cytotoxic and interstitial edema. Vasogenic cerebral edema is primarily a consequence of the increased blood–brain barrier permeability. Interstitial edema is due to diminished resorption of CSF at the level of the arachnoid granulations in the dural sinuses. The fibrinous exudate in the subarachnoid space interferes with the resorptive function of the arachnoid granulations. As resorption is obstructed, CSF dynamics are altered, and there is a transependymal movement of fluid from the ventricular system into the brain parenchyma.[1] One of the earliest and most frequent findings on computed tomography (CT) in children with bacterial meningitis is that of increased CSF volume in the ventricular and subarachnoid spaces.[2-4] An additional contributing factor to interstitial edema is an increased CSF outflow resistance due to the accumulation of a purulent exudate in the basal cisterns. Cytotoxic edema develops secondary to swelling of the cellular elements of the brain as a result of toxic factors released from neutrophils and bacteria. The hyponatremia which occurs secondary to the secretion of antidiuretic hormone also contributes to the pathogenesis of cytotoxic edema, by producing hypotonicity of extracellular fluid and increasing the permeability of the brain to water.

In both experimental models of meningitis and in clinical studies, it has been shown that, during the very early stages of meningitis, cerebral blood flow is increased and is associated with an increase in cerebral blood volume.[2,5-7]

An increase in the intracranial pressure (ICP) is significant inasmuch as it affects cerebral perfusion pressure (CPP). Cerebral perfusion pressure is defined as the difference between the mean arterial pressure and the intracranial pressure (CPP=MAP−ICP). A CPP of less than 40 torr is generally associated with cerebral ischemia. In studies in children with bacterial meningitis utilizing continuous ICP monitoring, it has been demonstrated that the decrease in CPP, particularly for those children who did not survive, was related less to systemic hypotension than to increased ICP.[2,8-10] Intracranial pressure is maximally elevated within the first 24–48 hours of hospitalization.[2,11,12]

References

1. Kaplan SL, Fishman MA. Supportive therapy for bacterial meningitis. *Pediatr Infect Dis J* 1987; **6:** 670–7.
2. Ashwal S, Tomasi L, Schneider S, Perkin R, Thompson J. Bacterial meningitis in children: pathophysiology and treatment. *Neurology* 1992; **42:** 739–48.
3. Stovring J, Snyder RD. Computed tomography in childhood bacterial meningitis. *J Pediatr* 1980; **96:** 820–3.

4. Cabral DA, Flodmark O, Farrell K, Speert DP. Prospective study of computed tomography in acute bacterial meningitis. *J Pediatr* 1987; **111:** 201–5.
5. Pfister HW, Koedel U, Haberi RL, et al. Microvascular changes during the early phase of experimental bacterial meningitis. *J Cereb Blood Flow Metab* 1990; **10:** 914–22.
6. Tureen J. Cerebral blood flow and metabolism in experimental meningitis. *Pediatr Infect Dis J* 1989; **8:** 917–19.
7. Tauber MG. Brain edema, intracranial pressure and cerebral blood flow in bacterial meningitis. *Pediatr Infect Dis J* 1989; **8:** 915–17.
8. Goiten KJ, Tamir I. Cerebral perfusion pressure in central nervous system infections of infancy and childhood. *J Pediatr* 1983; **103:** 40–3.
9. Gaussorgues P, Guerin C, Boyer F, et al. Intracranial hypertension in comatose bacterial meningitis. *Presse Med* 1987; **16:** 1420–3.
10. Rebaud P, Berthier JC, Hartemann E, Floret D. Intracranial pressure in childhood central nervous system infections. *Intensive Care Med* 1988; **14:** 522–5.
11. Dodge PR, Swartz MN. Bacterial meningitis: a review of selected aspects. II. Special neurologic problems, post meningitis complications and clinicopathological correlations. *N Engl J Med* 1965; **272:** 954–60.
12. McMenamin JB, Volpe JJ. Bacterial meningitis in infancy: effects on intracranial pressure and cerebral blood flow velocity. *Neurology* 1984; **34:** 500–4.

8. *Abnormalities in cerebral blood flow in bacterial meningitis are due to increased intracranial pressure, loss of autoregulation, narrowing of large arteries at the base of the brain, vasculitis, and thrombosis of cerebral arteries, veins and major sinuses*

Although there is an early hyperemia in bacterial meningitis, soon thereafter, cerebral blood flow begins to decrease and this contributes significantly to severe neurologic complications. Paulson et al.[1] measured a decreased regional cerebral blood flow using an intra-arterial injection of xenon (^{133}Xe) in five patients with pneumococcal meningitis. Tureen et al.[2] demonstrated a loss of cerebrovascular autoregulation in experimental pneumococcal meningitis in rabbits due to induced changes in systemic blood pressure. Cerebrovascular autoregulation normally occurs through dilatation or constriction of cerebral resistance vessels in response to alterations in cerebral perfusion pressure, due to either changes in the mean arterial blood pressure or changes in intracranial pressure.[2] Paulson et al. demonstrated loss of autoregulation in 6 of 10 adults with bacterial (pneumococcal and meningococcal) meningitis.

A loss of cerebral autoregulation implies that cerebral blood flow increases when the systemic blood pressure is raised and decreases when systemic blood pressure is lowered. A loss of cerebral autoregulation has not consistently been demonstrated in children with bacterial meningitis but rather local areas of markedly decreased cerebral blood flow due to inflammation or thrombosis of cerebral arteries, veins and sinuses have accounted for the majority of the cerebral infarctions. It is also possible that cerebral infarction is due not only to loss of cerebral autoregulation but also to a combination of local vascular pathology, raised intracranial pressure and loss of autoregulation.[3,4] Ischemia is not the only consequence of loss of cerebral autoregulation. With loss of cerebral autoregulation, changes in cerebral blood flow will contribute significantly to acute changes in intracranial pressure. As such, increased cerebral blood flow will further increase intracranial pressure.

One of the earliest reports of cerebrovascular complications during bacterial meningitis is the report of Lyons and Leeds (1967) of a 6-month-old infant who was admitted to the hospital with a left hemiplegia. *Haemophilus influenzae* was cultured from the blood and cerebrospinal fluid. Cerebral angiography demonstrated a considerable narrowing in caliber of the supraclinoid portions of the internal carotid arteries (ICA) bilaterally. The infant died 13 days after admission, and at autopsy the carotid arteries were thickened bilaterally and their lumens were greatly narrowed. The angiographic changes were attributed to severe stenosis of the arteries produced by the surrounding purulent exudate and the associated vasculitis with involvement of the intima.[5,6]

In a review of the angiographic abnormalities in 10 children ranging in age from 18 days to 4 years 11 months, with bacterial meningitis (*H. influenzae* in 7 cases, and group B streptococcus, *Streptococcus pneumoniae*, *Escherichia coli* in 1 case each), stenosis and/or occlusion of the major blood vessels at the base of the brain involving the supraclinoid portion of the ICA, and the proximal portion of the middle cerebral artery (MCA) and/or the anterior cerebral artery (ACA) was documented in all 10 cases.[6] The cerebrovascular complications, which were heralded by the onset of a neurologic deficit, occurred in the majority of patients on the third and fourth day of their illness, despite appropriate treatment for bacterial meningitis.

Cerebral angiography was performed in 27 adults with bacterial meningitis: in 21 because of a focal neurologic deficit on examination, a focal abnormality on cranial computed tomography (CT), or both; in 3 because of clinical signs of herniation; and in 3 individuals who had persistent coma without a defined etiology (despite 3 days of antimicrobial therapy). Angiography was performed between day 1 and day 21 after the onset of disease (median, day 3). Angiographic abnormalities were identified in 13 of the 27 patients and are as follows:

1. arterial narrowing of the major arteries at the base of the brain, including the supraclinoid portion of the ICA, the cerebellar arteries and the posterior cerebral arteries;
2. vessel wall irregularities of the medium-sized arteries with narrowed and ectatic segments, and obstructions of branches of the middle cerebral artery;
3. focal abnormal parenchymal blush;
4. thrombosis of the major sinuses and thrombophlebitis of the cerebral cortical veins.

Seven of the 13 patients with angiographically documented cerebrovascular complications had cerebral infarctions on cranial CT at the time of angiography. The prognosis of bacterial meningitis in the patients with cerebrovascular complications was extremely poor. Six of these patients died, 1 was in a persistent vegetative state, 4 had moderate or slight neuro-logic disability, and only 2 patients recovered completely.[7]

The most common cerebrovascular complication of bacterial meningitis appears to be narrowing of the large arteries at the base of the brain. The arterial narrowing is due to several etiologies, including:

1. encroachment on the vessel by the purulent exudate in the subarachnoid spaces and in the cisterns;
2. infiltration of the arterial wall by inflammatory cells with intimal thickening;
3. subintimal infiltration of the arterial wall (vasculitis);
4. vasospasm.[6–10]

The presence of cortical vein thrombosis in bacterial meningitis was found as early as 1948 in autopsy cases by Adams et al.,[10] and 1965 by Dodge and Schwartz,[8] and can be the cause of bland or hemorrhagic cerebral infarction, seizure activity or coma in the course of this infection.

References

1. Paulson OB, Brodersen P, Hansen EL, Kristensen HS. Regional cerebral blood flow, cerebral metabolic rate of oxygen, and cerebrospinal fluid acid–base variables in patients with acute meningitis and with acute encephalitis. *Acta Med Scand* 1974; **196:** 191–8.
2. Tureen JH, Dworkin RJ, Kennedy SL, Sachdena M, Sande MA. Loss of cerebrovascular autoregulation in experimental meningitis in rabbits. *J Clin Invest* 1990; **85:** 577–81.
3. Ashwal S, Tomasi L, Schneider S, Perkin R, Thompson J. Bacterial meningitis in children: pathophysiology and treatment. *Neurology* 1992; **42:** 739–48.
4. Snyder RD, Stovring J, Cushing A, Davis LE, Hardy TI. Cerebral infarction in childhood bacterial meningitis. *J Neurol Neurosurg Psychiatry* 1981; **44:** 581–5.
5. Lyons EL, Leeds NE. The angiographic demonstration of arterial vascular disease in purulent meningitis. *Radiology* 1967; **88:** 935–8.
6. Igarashi M, Gilmartin RC, Gerald B, Wilburn F, Jabbour JT. Cerebral arteritis and bacterial meningitis. *Arch Neurol* 1984; **41:** 531–5.
7. Pfister HW, Borasio GD, Dirnagl U, Bauer M, Einhaupl KM. Cerebrovascular complications of bacterial meningitis in adults. *Neurology* 1992; **42:** 1497–504.
8. Dodge PR, Swartz MN. Bacterial meningitis: a review of selected aspects. *N Engl J Med* 1965; **272:** 1003–10.
9. Raimondi AJ, DiRocco C. The physiopathogenetic basis for the angiographic diagnosis of bacterial infections of the brain and its coverings in children. *Childs Brain* 1979; **5:** 1–13.
10. Adams RD, Kubik CS, Bonner FJ. The clinical and pathological aspects of influenzal meningitis. *Arch Pediatr* 1948; **65:** 354–76, 408–41.

3
Clinical Presentation of Bacterial Meningitis

9. The triad of headache, fever and stiff neck is the classic presentation of bacterial meningitis

The characteristic symptoms and signs of bacterial meningitis are headache, fever, nuchal rigidity, photophobia, vomiting and lethargy or an altered level of consciousness, but the clinical symptoms and signs may vary depending on the age of the patient (Table 9.1) and the duration of illness prior to presentation.

Table 9.1   The clinical presentation of bacterial meningitis by age group

Neonates and infants
Fever (50%)
Lethargy
Poor feeding
Irritability
Vomiting and diarrhea
Apnea
Seizures
Bulging anterior fontanel

Children and adults
Fever
Headache
Photophobia
Nuchal rigidity
Lethargy, stupor, confusion or coma
Seizures
Focal neurologic deficits
Nausea and vomiting

Older adults
Fever
Headache
Nuchal rigidity
Confusion or coma
Seizures

The symptoms and signs of bacterial meningitis in the neonate are often subtle and typically nonspecific and include fever (50%), lethargy, poor feeding, respiratory distress, irritability, vomiting and diarrhea, seizures (40%) and a bulging fontanel (30%).[1] Very-low-birth-weight and premature infants are at risk for late-onset sepsis and meningitis and, in these infants, the initial clinical presentation of meningitis is nonspecific and typical of sepsis. The predominant findings are apnea, bradycardia, abdominal distention and seizures.[2] Fever is present at some time during the illness in most infants with meningitis, but may not be present in the neonate and premature infant. The temperature response to invasive bacterial infection in the premature infant is often that of hypothermia rather than fever.[3]

In children and adults, the typical symptoms and signs of bacterial meningitis are fever, headache, vomiting, photophobia, nuchal rigidity and lethargy, confusion or coma. Meningitis in children typically presents as either a subacute infection that gets progressively worse over several days and was preceded by an upper respiratory tract infection or otitis media, or as an acute fulminant illness that develops rapidly in a few hours. The clinical presentation of bacterial meningitis may be altered slightly by prior antibiotic therapy in the pediatric age group. Children who have been treated with oral antibiotics prior to the diagnosis of meningitis may have a longer duration of symptoms, more physical findings of ENT infections and less of a temperature elevation than children who have not had prior oral antibiotic therapy.[4] In adults, an upper respiratory infection frequently precedes the development of meningeal symptoms and should be sought after in the history. The clinical presentation of meningitis in an older adult consists of fever and either confusion, stupor or coma. The presentation of bacterial meningitis in an immunocompromised patient may be either suggestive of a mild infectious illness with headache and fever, or that of a fulminant illness presenting with coma and nuchal rigidity.

References

1. Feigin RD, McCracken GH, Klein JO. Diagnosis and management of meningitis. *Pediatr Infect Dis J* 1992; **11**: 785–814.
2. Perlman JM, Rollins N, Sanchez PJ. Late-onset meningitis in sick, very-low-birth-weight infants. *Am J Dis Child* 1992; **146**: 1297–301.
3. Bell WE. Bacterial meningitis in children: selected aspects. *Pediatr Clin North Amer* 1992; **39**: 651–68.
4. Rothrock SG, Green SM, Wren J, Letai D, Daniel-Underwood L, Pillar E. Pediatric bacterial meningitis: is prior antibiotic therapy associated with an altered clinical presentation? *Ann Emerg Med* 1992; **21**(2): 146–52.

10.   *The classic sign of bacterial meningitis is meningismus*

A stiff neck is the pathognomonic sign of meningeal irritation. Nuchal rigidity is present when the neck resists passive flexion (Fig. 10.1). Kernig's sign and Brudzinski's signs are also classic signs of meningeal irritation.

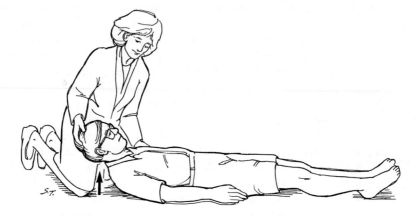

Fig. 10.1   Nuchal rigidity, a classic sign of meningitis, is present when the neck resists passive flexion.

Kernig's sign is elicited with the patient in the supine position. The thigh is flexed on the abdomen, with the knee flexed. Attempts to passively extend the leg elicit pain when meningeal irritation is present. The sign as originally described by Kernig, however, required the patient to be in the seated position (Fig. 10.2). Kernig noted that attempts to extend the knee, while the

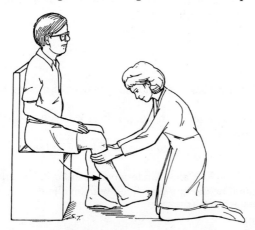

Fig. 10.2   Kernig's sign of meningeal irritation can be elicited with the patient in a seated or supine position, and is positive when attempts to extend the leg elicit pain, limiting the extension of the leg so that a "contracture of the extremities" is maintained.

patient was seated, were met with resistance in the presence of meningitis so that a "contracture of the extremities" was maintained.[1,2] Jozef Brudzinski described at least five different meningeal signs. His best known sign, the nape of the neck sign, is elicited with the patient in the supine position, and is positive when passive flexion of the neck results in spontaneous flexion of the hips and knees (Fig. 10.3).[3]

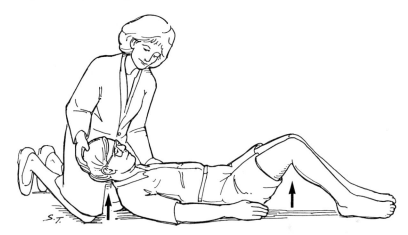

Fig. 10.3   Brudzinski's sign is elicited with the patient in the supine position, and is positive when passive flexion of the neck results in flexion of the hips and knees.

The differential diagnosis of neck stiffness in an acutely ill individual is as follows:

1. meningitis;
2. subarachnoid hemorrhage;
3. raised intracranial pressure with impending cerebellar tonsillar herniation;
4. infratentorial space-occupying mass lesion (i.e. cerebellar hematoma or abscess);
5. carcinomatous or leukemic meningeal infiltration;
6. neuroleptic malignant syndrome.[4]

Neck stiffness is sometimes difficult to interpret in the elderly individual. In this age group, resistance to passive movement of the neck may be due to meningitis, cervical spondylosis, parkinsonism or paratonic rigidity ("gegenhalten"). When neck stiffness is due to meningitis, the neck resists flexion but can usually be passively rotated from side to side. When neck stiffness is due to cervical spondylosis, parkinsonism or paratonic rigidity, any passive movement of the neck (lateral rotation, extension or flexion) meets with resistance.

References

1. Kernig VM. Ueber ein Krankheits symptom der acuten meningitis. *St Petersburg Medizinische Wochenschrift* 1882; **7**: 398.
2. Verghese A, Gallemore G. Kernig's and Brudzinski's signs revisited. *Rev Infect Dis* 1987; **9**: 1187–92.
3. Feigin RD, McCracken GH, Klein JO. Diagnosis and management of meningitis. *Pediatr Infect Dis J* 1992; **11**: 785–814.
4. Wildemann B, Dal Pan G. Neck stiffness and headache. In: Hacke W (ed.), *Neurocritical Care*. Berlin: Springer-Verlag, 1994; 285–91.

11.   Expect seizures in the first few days of meningitis

Seizures occur in 40% of patients with bacterial meningitis and typically occur in the first week of illness. The etiology of seizure activity can be attributed to either one or a combination of the following:

1. fever;
2. focal arterial ischemia or infarction;
3. cortical venous thrombosis with hemorrhage;
4. hyponatremia;
5. subdural effusion producing a mass effect;
6. antimicrobial agents.

The majority of seizures have a focal onset, suggesting that focal ischemia from cerebrovascular disease is a major cause of seizure activity in bacterial meningitis. Hughlings Jackson in 1876, Gowers in 1885, Dunham in 1916 and Dodge in 1954 described a definite association between cerebrovascular disease and convulsions,[1] but it was not until recently that the incidence and nature of cerebrovascular disease in bacterial meningitis was closely investigated[2] and a relationship established between cerebrovascular disease and convulsions in bacterial meningitis.

Seizure activity that has a focal onset is most likely to be the result of focal cerebrovascular disease due to the infection, or focal edema or mass effect from an expanding subdural effusion. Generalized seizure activity and status epilepticus are due to fever, hyponatremia, anoxia from decreased cerebral perfusion due to increased intracranial pressure, spread from a focal onset to a generalized tonic–clonic convulsion or toxicity from antimicrobial agents (imipenem, penicillin).

References

1. Richardson EP, Dodge PR. Epilepsy in cerebral vascular disease. *Epilepsia* 1954; **3**: 49–71.

2. Pfister HW, Borasio GD, Dirnagl U, Bauer M, Einhaupl KM. Cerebrovascular complications of bacterial meningitis in adults. *Neurology* 1992; **42:** 1497–504.

12. *Raised intracranial pressure is an expected complication of bacterial meningitis*

In the presence of raised intracranial pressure, any one or a combination of the following clinical signs may develop:

1. an altered level of consciousness;
2. the Cushing reflex – bradycardia, hypertension and irregular respirations;[1]
3. dilated, nonreactive pupil;
4. unilateral or bilateral cranial nerve VI palsies;
5. papilledema;
6. neck stiffness;
7. hiccups;
8. projective vomiting;
9. decerebrate posturing (Fig. 12.1).

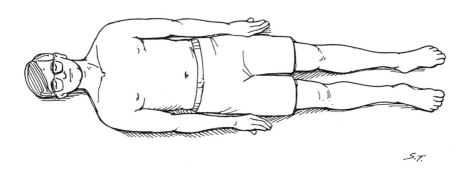

Fig. 12.1   In decerebrate or "abnormal extensor" posturing, the arms are adducted, rigidly extended and hyperpronated, and the legs are rigidly extended with plantar flexion of the feet.

The presence of raised intracranial pressure (ICP) can be determined by obtaining an opening pressure at the time of the initial lumbar puncture. The range of values for normal opening pressure as measured from a lumbar puncture with a patient in the lateral supine position are listed in Table 12.1.[2,3]

Opening pressure should be measured in the lateral supine position because the sitting position does not allow for accurate measurement of CSF pressure. It is estimated that CSF pressure obtained from the lumbar interspace with the patient in a sitting position is about 150 mm higher than CSF pressure obtained with the patient in the lateral recumbent position.

Table 12.1   Normal range of opening pressure by age group with the patient in the lateral recumbent position.

Age group	CSF pressure (mmH$_2$O)
Infants and children to 6 years of age	10–120
Children and adults	10–180
Obese adults	≤250

Source: Fishman (1992);[2] Corbett and Mehta (1983).[3]

The needle should be inserted in the L3–4, L4–5, or L5–S1 interspaces (Fig. 12.2). Insertion of the needle at higher levels should be avoided because the termination of the spinal cord, the conus medullaris, is at either the L1–2

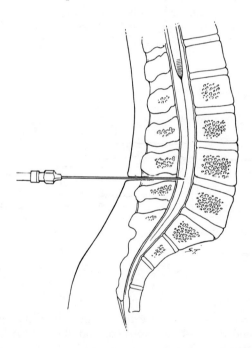

Fig. 12.2   Technique of lumbar puncture. The patient is placed in the lateral recumbent position with the neck and knees flexed. A 22- or 20-gauge needle is inserted below the termination of the spinal cord (the L1–2 or L2–3 interspace) in the L3–4, L4–5, or L5–S1 interspaces.

interspace or the L2–3 interspace. A spuriously elevated opening pressure may be obtained due to: failure to position the patient properly; abdominal muscle straining which elevates the central venous pressure; or obesity. The patient should be as comfortable as possible with the knees flexed to the chest and the neck flexed.

To assess opening pressure accurately in an infant, the technique of the lumbar puncture should be modified slightly from that which is routinely performed for an older child or adult. If the child's head is held very tightly flexed, CSF may not be obtained. It is recommended that the child's head be held in midflexion.[2] The depth of the needle for lumbar puncture should be no greater than 2.5 cm in small infants.[2,4]

When clinical signs of elevated ICP are present, this should be monitored by an ICP monitoring device. Elevated ICP can cause death by brainstem compression and cardiopulmonary arrest, and produces neurologic morbidity by decreasing cerebral blood flow with resultant cerebral ischemia.[5] Normal ICP, as measured by an ICP monitoring device, is less than 10 mmHg. Sustained elevations in ICP above 15 mmHg should be treated. The treatment of elevated intracranial pressure is outlined in Table 12.2.[6,7]

Table 12.2   Treatment of raised intracranial pressure in bacterial meningitis

---

1. Elevate the head of the bed 30°. Keep the head in the midline position
2. Hyperventilation to maintain $PaCO_2$ between 25–33 mmHg
3. Mannitol
   1.0 g/kg bolus injection and then 0.25–0.5 g/kg every 3–5 hours to achieve a serum osmolarity of 295–320 mOsm/L
4. Dexamethasone 0.15 mg/kg every 6 hours
5. Pentobarbital coma
   Loading dose: 5–10 mg/kg intravenously given at a rate of 1 mg/kg/min
   Maintenance dose: 1–3 mg/kg/h. Therapy can be titrated to achieve a therapeutic serum level of 25–40 mg/L or a burst-suppression pattern on electroencephalogram (EEG)
6. Thiopental (1–5 mg/kg) or lidocaine (75–100 mg) prior to endotracheal suctioning or chest physiotherapy

---

Source: Dacey (1987);[7] Ropper(1993).[6]

References

1. Cushing H. Concerning a definite regulatory mechanism of the vaso-motor centre which controls blood pressure during cerebral compression. *Johns Hopkins Hosp Bull* 1901; **12:** 290–2.
2. Fishman RA. Examination of the cerebrospinal fluid: techniques and complications. In: Fishman RA (ed.), *Cerebrospinal Fluid in Diseases of the Nervous System.* Philadelphia: W.B. Saunders, 1992; 157–82.
3. Corbett JJ, Mehta MP. Cerebrospinal fluid pressure in normal obese subjects and patients with pseudotumor cerebri. *Neurology* 1983; **33**(10): 1386–8.
4. Bonadio WA, Smith DS, Metron M, DeWitz B. Estimating lumbar puncture depth in children. *N Engl J Med* 1988; **319:** 952–3.
5. Ropper AH, Rockoff MA. Physiology and clinical aspects of raised intracranial pressure. In: Ropper AH (ed.), *Neurological and Neurosurgical Intensive Care.* New York: Raven Press, 1993; 11–27.
6. Ropper AH. Treatment of intracranial hypertension. In: Ropper AH (ed.),

Neurological and Neurosurgical Intensive Care. New York: Raven Press, 1993; 29–52.
7. Dacey RG. Monitoring and treating increased intracranial pressure. *Pediatr Infect Dis J* 1987; **6:** 1161–3.

13.   There is a risk of cerebral herniation in bacterial meningitis that is independent of lumbar puncture

Patients with bacterial meningitis are at risk for cerebral herniation. In one series of 302 infants and children with acute bacterial meningitis, cerebral herniation occurred in 18 cases (6%). Eleven of the 18 cases of cerebral herniation had meningitis due to *Haemophilus influenzae* type b (Hib), and 7 had meningitis due to *Streptococcus pneumoniae*. In all 18 patients, cerebral herniation happened within 8 hours of admission, and in 8 cases cerebral herniation occurred within 30 minutes of admission. Three of the patients with this complication died, and 4 of the 15 patients who survived had severe neurologic deficits at the time of discharge from the hospital. In the 8 patients who developed clinical signs of cerebral herniation within 30 minutes of admission to the hospital, a possible relationship to lumbar puncture was suggested. In each case the amount of CSF removed was approximately 2–3 ml. One of the patients developed respiratory arrest, and fixed and dilated pupils immediately following lumbar puncture; an autopsy was not obtained.[1]

Dodge and Swartz[2] addressed the issue of the relationship of cerebral herniation to lumbar puncture in their classic paper on bacterial meningitis. In this series of 29 patients dying with acute bacterial meningitis, there were 3 cases of temporal lobe herniation and 7 cases of cerebellar herniation. Death from herniation followed lumbar puncture immediately or within 2 hours in 3 cases. The difficulty in attributing these episodes of cerebral herniation to the procedure itself is emphasized by one of the patients with meningococcal meningitis who died of medullary compression from a cerebellar pressure cone before lumbar puncture.

In 279 episodes of community-acquired meningitis, there were 8 cases of autopsy-proven cerebral herniation. All had temporal-lobe herniation; 4 also had cerebellar herniation. All had cerebral edema; 2 also had dural sinus or cortical vein thrombosis. This series may have included some of the patients described in the Dodge and Swartz series.[2] The amount of time between lumbar puncture and cerebral herniation is not documented except to state that clinical signs of cerebral herniation developed within a period of time ranging from several minutes to several hours after a lumbar puncture.[3]

In a prospective study of 86 patients with bacterial meningitis between the ages of 15 and 87, cerebral herniation occurred in 7 patients during the acute phase of the illness. This was due to cerebral edema in 4 patients, angiographically documented sinus venous thrombosis in 2 patients, and hydrocephalus in one patient.[4]

In a retrospective study to determine whether the incidence of cerebral herniation was increased immediately after lumbar puncture, the medical records of 445 children (aged 1 month and older) with bacterial meningitis were reviewed. Cerebral herniation occurred in 19 (4%) of the 445 children. Herniation occurred within 3 hours of lumbar puncture in 8 children. Of these children, 3 had signs suggesting impending herniation at the time of the procedure (these children were comatose and unresponsive to pain at the time of lumbar puncture), cerebral herniation had occurred previously in 1 (this child had had dilatation of one pupil before being paralyzed and ventilated), 1 child with hypotonic cerebral palsy was hard to assess, and 1 child had decerebrate posturing at the time of the lumbar puncture. Six of the 19 episodes of herniation occurred before lumbar puncture or in a child that did not undergo lumbar puncture.[5,6]

The clinical signs of cerebral herniation are as follows:

1. coma;
2. unilateral or bilateral fixed and dilated pupils;
3. decorticate or decerebrate posture;
4. Cheyne–Stokes respirations, hyperventilation, apnea or respiratory arrest;
5. loss of oculocephalic response or fixed oculomotor deviation.[1]

The risk of cerebral herniation from acute bacterial meningitis is approximately 6–8%. Focal or diffuse cerebral edema is the most likely etiology; however, hydrocephalus and dural sinus or cortical vein thrombosis may also cause herniation. The role of lumbar puncture as a causative factor for cerebral herniation has been debated for at least 30 years, and remains unclear. When the possibility of increased intracranial pressure exists, lumbar puncture should be performed with a 22-gauge needle, 30–60 minutes after 1 g/kg mannitol has been administered intravenously. The removal of only 3–5 mL of CSF is recommended for analysis.

References

1. Horwitz SJ, Boxerbaum B, O'Bell J. Cerebral herniation in bacterial meningitis in childhood. *Ann Neurol* 1980; **7**: 524–8.
2. Dodge PR, Swartz MN. Bacterial meningitis - a review of selected aspects; special neurologic problems, postmeningitic complications and clinicopathologic correlations. *N Engl J Med* 1965; **272**: 954–60.
3. Durand ML, Calderwood SB, Weber DJ, Miller SI, Southwick FS, Caviness VS, Swartz MN. Acute bacterial meningitis in adults. *N Engl J Med* 1993; **328**: 21–8.
4. Pfister HW, Feiden W, Einhaupl KM. The spectrum of complications during bacterial meningitis in adults: results of a prospective clinical study. *Arch Neurol* 1993; **50**: 575–81.
5. Rennick G, Shann F, deCampo J. Cerebral herniation during bacterial meningitis in children. *Br Med J* 1993; **306**: 953–5.
6. Jones SW, Webb D. Cerebral herniation in bacterial meningitis. *Br Med J* 1993; **306**: 1413.

14.   *Focal intracranial mass lesions, herpes simplex virus encephalitis and subarachnoid hemorrhage should be included in the differential diagnosis of bacterial meningitis*

The differential diagnosis of headache, fever, focal neurologic symptoms and/or an altered level of consciousness is the following:

1. herpes simplex virus (HSV) encephalitis;
2. focal infectious mass lesions;
3. subarachnoid hemorrhage;
4. Lyme disease;
5. rickettsial infections;
6. fungal meningitis;
7. neuroleptic malignant syndrome.

Herpes simplex virus has a predilection for the inferior frontal and medial temporal lobes; therefore, a change in mentation or behavior is a common manifestation of HSV encephalitis. The usual clinical presentation of HSV encephalitis includes:

1. fever;
2. headache;
3. confusion or a change in behavior;
4. new onset seizure activity which is frequently focal in nature;
5. focal neurologic deficit, such as aphasia, hemiparesis, etc.

Examination of the CSF demonstrates a lymphocytic pleocytosis, the presence of red blood cells, an elevated protein concentration and a slight xanthochromia. The polymerase chain reaction technique to detect HSV DNA in the CSF is a highly sensitive and specific test that is becoming more readily available, and should be performed whenever possible. A four-fold rise in HSV antibodies is helpful to confirm the diagnosis; however, this takes 1–4 weeks, and is not particularly useful in the acute situation. The electroencephalogram (EEG) may confirm the temporal lobe localization of the infection by demonstrating periodic spike and sharp wave activity, which initially arises from one temporal region but may become bilateral after several days. Magnetic resonance scan is often positive demonstrating areas of increased signal intensity in the frontotemporal areas on T_2-weighted imaging.

Focal infectious mass lesions have a clinical presentation similar to meningitis. The most common symptom of a brain abscess is a hemicranial or generalized headache with focal neurologic deficits and/or new onset focal or generalized seizure activity. Fever is present in 50% of patients. A subdural empyema presents as a headache which becomes increasingly more severe followed by an alteration in the level of consciousness. Focal neurologic deficits are present in 80–90% of patients. Fever is typically present. The classic presentation of an intracranial epidural abscess is an unrelenting hemicranial headache with fever. A neuroimaging procedure is indicated prior to lumbar puncture if a focal infectious mass lesion is suspected.

The classic presentation of a subarachnoid hemorrhage is the explosive onset of a severe headache, or a sudden transient loss of consciousness followed by a severe headache. Nuchal rigidity and vomiting are frequently present. Computed tomography (CT) may demonstrate blood in the basal cisterns. If the CT scan is normal, an examination of the CSF is indicated. Red blood cells are present in the CSF within minutes of the rupture of an intracranial aneurysm. The appearance of red blood cells in the CSF necessitates distinguishing between a bloody tap and a subarachnoid hemorrhage. When bloody fluid is obtained at lumbar puncture, the fluid should be collected in at least three separate tubes. In a traumatic puncture, the fluid typically clears between the first and the third tubes. In a subarachnoid hemorrhage, the fluid will remain blood-tinged in all three tubes. A sample of the bloody CSF should be centrifuged. In a traumatic puncture, the supernatant is colorless, whereas in subarachnoid hemorrhage the supernatant is yellow (xanthochromic). It takes at least 2–4 hours for xanthochromia to appear, and it may take as long as 12 hours.[1]

The predominant symptom of meningitis due to Lyme disease is headache. This may be accompanied by facial or other cranial neuropathies and/or peripheral neuropathies. Examination of the CSF demonstrates a mononuclear pleocytosis, a mild elevation in the protein concentration and a normal glucose concentration. The diagnosis is made by the demonstration of the intrathecal production of anti-*Borrelia burgdorferi* antibodies. The duration and severity of neurologic symptoms are much longer in Lyme disease than would be expected for acute bacterial meningitis. The characteristic skin lesion of Lyme disease, erythema chronicum migrans, may precede the symptoms of meningitis.

Rocky Mountain Spotted Fever (RMSF) is characterized by headache, fever, rash and confusion or an altered level of consciousness. The rash of RMSF consists of 1–5 mm pink macules which are most often first noticed on the wrist and ankles, and then spread centrally to the chest, face and abdomen. After a few days, the macules turn dark red or purple. Diagnosis can be made by biopsy of the skin lesions and staining of the specimen with fluorescent antibodies to *Rickettsia rickettsii*.

Fungal meningitis, and especially cryptococcal meningitis, may present as an acute illness with fever, headache, and an altered sensorium. Examination of the CSF demonstrates a lymphocytic pleocytosis with an elevated protein concentration and a decreased glucose concentration. The latex agglutination test for the cryptococcal antigen is a highly sensitive and specific test. The India ink stain is more frequently positive in HIV-infected individuals than in HIV-negative individuals.

The characteristic signs of neuroleptic malignant syndrome are fever (as high as 41°C), generalized lead-pipe rigidity, tachycardia, fluctuating level of consciousness (from agitation to stupor and coma), blood pressure instability,

Table 14.1   The clinical presentation of diseases in the differential diagnosis of acute bacterial meningitis

Disease	Clinical presentation
Herpes simplex virus encephalitis	Fever, confusion, change in behavior Headache New-onset focal or generalized seizure activity Focal neurologic deficits
Brain abscess	Hemicranial or generalized headache Focal neurologic deficits New-onset focal or generalized seizure activity ± Fever
Subdural empyema	Severe headache localized to the side of the subdural infection Altered level of consciousness Fever, chills, nuchal rigidity Focal neurologic deficits
Intracranial epidural abscess	Hemicranial headache Fever Recent history of sinusitis, mastoiditis or otitis media
Subarachnoid hemorrhage	Explosive onset of severe headache Vomiting Syncope Nuchal rigidity Altered level of consciousness Dilated, non-reactive pupil
Rocky Mountain spotted fever	Headache, fever Petechial rash Altered mental status
Lyme disease	History of tick bite and/or erythema chronicum migrans Facial nerve palsy
Cryptococcal meningitis	Fever, headache Skin lesions Cranial nerve palsies
Tuberculous meningitis	Headache, meningismus Confusion, coma, seizures
Neuroleptic malignant syndrome	Fever Generalized lead-pipe rigidity Fluctuating level of consciousness Autonomic instability

diaphoresis and tachypnea. A marked elevation in the serum creatine kinase concentration, usually exceeding 10,000 IU/L, and a leukocytosis of 15,000–30,000 cells/mm³ are common. A history of neuroleptic therapy is helpful when provided.

Table 14.1 lists the clinical presentations of diseases in the differential diagnosis of acute bacterial meningitis, and Table 14.2 lists the diagnostic studies that are useful to differentiate acute bacterial meningitis from the diseases in the differential diagnosis.

Table 14.2   Diagnostic studies to differentiate acute bacterial meningitis from the diseases in the differential diagnosis

Disease	Diagnostic study
Herpes simplex virus encephalitis	*CSF* – lymphocytic pleocytosis, red blood cells *MRI* – increased signal intensity on T_2-weighted images in temporal lobe(s) *EEG* – periodic spike and slow-wave activity in temporal lobe(s)
Brain abscess, subdural empyema, intracranial epidural abscess	Contrast-enhanced CT scan or gadolinium-enhanced T_1-weighted MRI
Subarachnoid hemorrhage	Non-contrast-enhanced CT scan may demonstrate blood in the basal cisterns *CSF* – red blood cells, xanthochromia
Rocky Mountain spotted fever	Biopsy skin lesions
Lyme disease	*CSF* – mononuclear pleocytosis and intrathecal anti-*Borrelia burgdorferi* antibody production *Serum* – Lyme serology
Cryptococcal meningitis	*CSF* – lymphocytic pleocytosis, positive cryptococcal antigen Biopsy skin lesions
Tuberculous meningitis	*CSF* – lymphocytic pleocytosis, acid-fast bacilli Purified protein derivative Chest X-ray
Neuroleptic malignant syndrome	*CSF* – normal Marked elevation in the serum CK Leukocytosis of 15,000–30,000 cells/mm³

CSF, cerebrospinal fluid; MRI, magnetic resonance imaging; EEG, electroencephalogram; CT, computed tomography; CK, creatine kinase.

References

1. Fishman RA. Composition of the cerebrospinal fluid. In: Fishman RA (ed.), *Cerebrospinal Fluid in Diseases of the Nervous System.* Philadelphia: W.B. Saunders, 1992; 183–252.

15.   *A lumbar puncture is not required in all instances of febrile seizures in childhood*

Febrile seizures are seizures in infancy or childhood, usually occurring between 3 months and 5 years of age, associated with fever but not due to central nervous system infectious diseases.[1,2] The estimated prevalence of febrile seizures is in the range of 2–5% of young children in the United States.[2,3] Seizures precipitated by fever in young children are the most common seizures of childhood.[4] There is a genetic predisposition to febrile convulsions. The average age of onset for febrile seizures is 18–22 months. Febrile seizures usually occur in the presence of an upper respiratory infection, otitis media, a gastrointestinal infection or roseola infantum. Central nervous system infectious diseases are excluded from this list by definition. A simple febrile seizure, by definition, occurs in association with fever and is of brief duration (<15 minutes), non-focal and non-repetitive.[1] A febrile convulsion is typically characterized by rhythmic clonic movements with tonic stiffening of the extremities, is associated with loss of consciousness, and is followed by a postictal period with unresponsiveness. In most instances of a benign febrile convulsion, the seizure has ended before the child is brought to medical attention.[2] Except in the young infant, in the absence of clinical signs of meningitis, the yield of a lumbar puncture is very low.

In one review of the results of lumbar puncture in 314 patients with febrile convulsions who had no clinical evidence of meningitis, the CSF demonstrated meningitis in 4 cases, 1 of which was bacterial, 3 of which were viral. All 4 children were 15 months of age or younger.[5]

As most children with a brief single febrile seizure have stopped seizing by the time they are brought to medical attention, an actively convulsing febrile child in the Emergency Room should have a lumbar puncture. It has been recommended that a lumbar puncture be performed in every child <2 years of age presenting with a febrile convulsion because of the difficulty in diagnosing meningitis in this age group by clinical signs alone.[6,7] By definition, a febrile seizure should be brief, single and non-focal; therefore, any febrile convulsion that is prolonged, repetitive or associated with focal neurologic deficits should be evaluated with a lumbar puncture. A child who has simply had a self-limited febrile seizure should be awake and alert following a brief postictal period; therefore, if the child remains lethargic or stuporous, lumbar puncture should be performed.[2] Close follow-up is recommended for all children presenting with a febrile convulsion to be certain that clinical signs of meningitis do not develop.

References

1. Consensus Statement. Febrile seizures: long-term management of children with fever-associated seizures. *Pediatrics* 1980; **66:** 1009–12.
2. Hirtz DG, Nelson KB. The natural history of febrile seizures. *Ann Rev Med* 1983; **34:** 453–71.
3. Nelson KB, Ellenberg JH. Prognosis in children with febrile seizures. *Pediatrics* 1978; **61:** 720–7.
4. Freeman JM. The best medicine for febrile seizures. *N Engl J Med* 1992; **327:** 1161–2.
5. Rutter N, Smales ORC. Role of routine investigations in children presenting with their first febrile convulsion. *Arch Dis Child* 1977; **52:** 188–91.
6. Wolf SM. Laboratory evaluation of the child with a febrile convulsion. *Pediatrics* 1978; **62:** 1074–6.
7. Ouellette EM. Managing febrile seizures. *Drug Ther* 1977; **2:** 37–9.

4
Cerebrospinal Fluid

16. *Meningitis can be diagnosed only by examination of the cerebrospinal fluid*

Analysis of the CSF is key to diagnosing meningitis. The majority of the CSF is formed in the choroid plexus of the lateral, third and fourth ventricles.

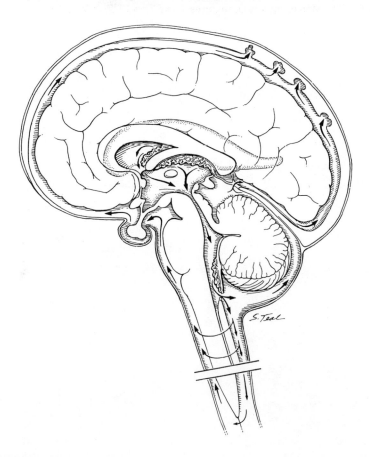

Fig. 16.1   Flow of cerebrospinal fluid from its formation in the choroid plexus of the lateral, third and fourth ventricles.

Cerebrospinal fluid flows out of the lateral ventricles through the foramina of Monro to the third ventricle; then, through the cerebral aqueduct to the fourth ventricle. It exits the fourth ventricle through the lateral foramina of Luschka and the foramen of Magendie into the subarachnoid space. The circulation of the CSF in the subarachnoid space is cephalad to the cerebral hemispheres and caudad to the cerebellum, brainstem and spinal cord (Fig. 16.1). Most of the CSF is absorbed into the venous system by the arachnoid villi and granulations, which are numerous projections of the arachnoid membrane located over the convexities of the brain that protrude into the lumina of the superior sagittal sinus.[1] The bulk of the CSF is formed in the choroid plexus, with the remainder being formed in extrachoroidal sites including the capillary bed of the brain, the ventricular ependyma, the Sylvian aqueduct and the subarachnoid pial surface.[2]

Heinrich Quincke developed the technique of lumbar puncture and described not only the analysis of the fluid but also the technique of recording the pressure with a manometer.[3]

The upper limit of normal CSF opening pressure with a patient in the lateral recumbent position is 110 mm of water in young infants, 150 mm of water in children, 180 mm of water in adults and 250 mm of water in obese adults. A normal upper range for CSF pressure with a patient in a seated position may be as high as 400 mm of water; therefore, this position is not recommended for obtaining an opening pressure.[2,4]

References

1. Fishman RA. Anatomical aspects of the cerebrospinal fluid. In: Fishman RA (ed.), *Cerebrospinal Fluid in Diseases of the Nervous System*. Philadelphia: W.B. Saunders, 1992; 7–21.
2. Bonadio WA. The cerebrospinal fluid: physiologic aspects and alterations associated with bacterial meningitis. *Pediatr Infect Dis J* 1992; **11**: 423–32.
3. Quincke H. Uber hydrocephalus, Verhandlungen des Congressus fur innere Medizin. Vol. 10. Wiesbaden: JF Bergman, 1891; 321.
4. Dougherty JM, Roth RM. Cerebral spinal fluid. *Emer Med Clin North Amer* 1986; **4**: 281–97.

17.   *Lumbar puncture should be part of the routine sepsis work-up in infants*

Lumbar puncture should be included in the diagnostic evaluation of infants with possible sepsis. Approximately 20–30% of cases of neonatal sepsis are complicated by bacterial meningitis.[1] The risk of iatrogenic meningeal infection due to lumbar puncture in a bacteremic infant is extremely small. In a recent review of 1880 lumbar punctures in infants, over an 8-year span, there was only one case of meningitis where it was possible that lumbar puncture during bacteremia may have caused meningeal infection.[1]

This raises the question: where does the fear of iatrogenic meningitis come from? The association between lumbar puncture and meningitis during bacteremia is based on the classic experimental work on the pathogenesis of meningitis by Petersdorf et al. and clinical reviews.[2,3] In experimental studies to define the pathogenesis of bacterial meningitis, Petersdorf et al.[2] postulated that the meninges were infected by the bloodstream. Prior to this investigation, experimental meningitis was produced in dogs by the introduction of pneumococci into the subarachnoid space through a burr hole. In the experiments of Petersdorf et al.,[2] pneumococci were injected into the saphenous vein. Cisternal puncture was performed within 2 minutes of intravenous administration of pneumococci. Only the animals subjected to cisternal puncture within 30 minutes of injection of pneumococci developed infection. Petersdorf concluded that in the dogs that developed meningitis, the bacteria entered the subarachnoid space through the small opening made at the time of cisternal puncture and therefore that trauma to the meninges in the form of cisternal puncture during pneumococcal bacteremia results in meningitis, provided sufficient numbers of pneumococci are in the bloodstream at the time of the cisternal puncture. Petersdorf et al.[2] also state that their data do not support the idea that suspected or documented bacteremia constitutes a contraindication to lumbar puncture and that "compared with the risk of missing the diagnosis of meningitis by omission of lumbar puncture, the chance of developing meningeal infection after the procedure is small."

Teele et al.[3] reviewed 277 episodes of bacteremia in 271 children. Ninety-one per cent of the children had a temperature greater than or equal to 38.9°C and 75% had a white cell count greater than or equal to 15,000/mL at the time of initial presentation. Forty-six children had a lumbar puncture performed. All CSF samples were normal. Five of these children were not treated with antimicrobial therapy. Two children were treated with oral antibiotics. Seven of the 46 children developed meningitis within 1–9 days after initial evaluation. All were under 1 year of age. The conclusion was made that there was a significant association between the lumbar puncture performed during bacteremia and the later development of bacterial meningitis in children under 1 year of age who received no initial antimicrobial therapy. However, there was a broad time range between the initial lumbar puncture and the subsequent development of meningitis (1–9 days) to attribute the meningitis to the lumbar puncture. It is more likely that meningitis developed as a complication of bacteremia in these seven children.

It should also be emphasized that a traumatic lumbar puncture performed in a bacteremic child who does not have meningitis could result in a positive CSF culture (from blood contaminating the spinal fluid) with a normal CSF chemistry and white cell count[1] and the erroneous interpretation that the child has meningitis.

Negative blood cultures do not rule out meningitis in the neonate. In one series, 15 of 28 (53%) newborns with bacterial meningitis on day one of life had negative blood cultures. Twenty-three of 47 (49%) older neonates (aged 8–28 days) with bacterial meningitis had negative blood cultures.[4] In other series, 6 of 39 (15%) neonates with bacterial meningitis had negative blood cultures.[5]

The lowest possible interspace should be used to perform lumbar puncture in infants because the conus medullaris extends even lower than L2–3 in infants.[6]

References

1. Hristeva L, Booy R, Bowler I, Wilkinson AR. Prospective surveillance of neonatal meningitis. *Arch Dis Child* 1993; **69:** 14–18.
2. Petersdorf RG, Swauner DR, Garcia M. Studies on the pathogenesis of meningitis. II. Development of meningitis during pneumococcal bacteremia. *J Clin Invest* 1962; **41:** 320–7.
3. Teele DW, Dashefsky B, Rakusan T, Klein JO. Meningitis after lumbar puncture in children with bacteremia. *N Engl J Med* 1981; **305:** 1079–81.
4. Shattuck KE, Chonmaitree T. The changing spectrum of neonatal meningitis over a fifteen-year period. *Clin Pediatr* 1992; **31**(3): 130–6.
5. Visser VE, Hall RT. Lumbar puncture in the evaluation of suspected neonatal sepsis. *J Pediatr* 1980; **96:** 1063–7.
6. Fishman RA. Examination of the cerebrospinal fluid: techniques and complications. In: Fishman RA (ed.), *Cerebrospinal Fluid in Diseases of the Nervous System.* Philadelphia: W.B. Saunders, 1992; 157–82.

18.   *A cranial CT scan is not always required before lumbar puncture is performed*

It has become fairly routine practice to perform a cranial computed tomography (CT) scan prior to lumbar puncture. This procedure, however, may delay therapy and is certainly not always necessary. The indications for cranial CT prior to lumbar puncture are as follows:

1. coma;
2. focal neurologic deficit;
3. papilledema;
4. a dilated, poorly reactive pupil;
5. signs of a posterior fossa mass lesion (cranial-nerve abnormalities, cerebellar deficit and a wide-based ataxic gait).

It has been said that the only urgent indication for lumbar puncture is the suspicion of bacterial meningitis.[1]

The most serious complication of lumbar puncture is uncal or cerebellar herniation or so-called "coning". The following clinical signs are suggestive of raised intracranial pressure and may have predictive value in determining which patients are at risk for herniation:

1. deterioration in the level of consciousness;
2. decerebrate or decorticate rigidity;
3. unilateral or bilateral fixed dilated pupils;
4. hemiparesis;
5. apnea or irregular respiration;
6. ocular motility abnormalities.[1]

Raised intracranial pressure is an expected complication of bacterial meningitis, and lumbar puncture is typically done in this setting. Once a CT scan has been obtained to exclude a focal intracranial mass lesion, lumbar puncture can usually be performed safely. When the presence of raised intracranial pressure is suspected, a bolus dose of mannitol 1 g/kg of body weight can be given intravenously and lumbar puncture performed 20 minutes later. Alternatively, the patient can be intubated and hyperventilated in addition to the use of intravenous mannitol. It is recommended that lumbar puncture be performed with a 22 gauge needle. Larger needles may create a rent in the dura that could lead to complications as CSF continues to leak from the intrathecal sac.

Lumbar puncture can be safely performed in patients with reactive pupils, normal optic discs and non-focal neurologic examinations. If the decision is made to delay lumbar puncture until a cranial CT scan can be obtained, broad-spectrum intravenous antimicrobial therapy should be initiated.

Can lumbar puncture be avoided altogether, with treatment of meningitis being initiated based on a clinical diagnosis alone? Lumbar puncture should be performed to:

1. confirm the diagnosis;
2. identify the organism;
3. test for antibiotic sensitivities;
4. rationalize the treatment of contacts in the case of meningococcal or *Haemophilus influenzae* meningitis.[1]

The diseases that have a clinical presentation very similar to bacterial meningitis are subarachnoid hemorrhage and herpes encephalitis. The CSF can help to differentiate these diseases from bacterial meningitis.

When obtaining CSF for analysis, it is important to remember that adults have approximately 150 mL of CSF, but infants and children have lower amounts ranging from 30–60 mL in the neonate to 100 mL in the adolescent.[2] The volume of CSF in a child of 4–13 years of age ranges from 65–140 mL with an average volume of 90 mL.[3] Approximately 10–12 mL of CSF should be withdrawn from the adult for analysis and the withdrawal of 3–5 mL is recommended in the neonate and child.[2]

Epidural and spinal subdural hematomas may complicate lumbar punctures that are performed in the setting of thrombocytopenia or a prolonged prothrombin time.

References

1. Addy DP. When not to do a lumbar puncture. *Arch Dis Child* 1987; **62:** 873–5.
2. Dougherty JM, Roth RM. Cerebral spinal fluid. *Emer Med Clin North Amer* 1986; **4:** 281–97.
3. Bonadio WA. The cerebrospinal fluid: physiologic aspects and alterations associated with bacterial meningitis. *Pediatr Infect Dis J* 1992; **11:** 423–32.

19.   *The presence of more than 5 WBCs/mm³ in CSF is abnormal in individuals 8 weeks of age and older*

The number of white blood cells (WBCs) in the CSF varies normaliy with age.

Newborn

The upper limit of normal value for CSF total WBC count is 22/mm³ in full term neonates, 30/mm³ in infants 0–8 weeks and 5/mm³ in those older than 8 weeks of age. In newborns, in normal uninfected CSF, about 60% of the cells are polymorphonuclear leukocytes and 40% are mononucleated cells.

Adults

In adults, in uninfected CSF the normal WBC count ranges from 0 to 5 mononuclear cells (lymphocytes and monocytes) per mm³. In normal uninfected CSF in the adult there should be no polymorphonuclear leukocytes; however, with the use of the cytocentrifuge, an occasional polymorphonuclear leukocyte may be seen. If the total WBC count is <5, the presence of a single polymorphonuclear leukocyte may be considered normal.[1–3]

When the spinal tap has been traumatic, the clinician is faced with the dilemma whether the CSF pleocytosis is real or whether the WBCs were introduced by the spinal tap itself. Blood is introduced into the CSF during lumbar puncture when the spinal needle passes through the subarachnoid space and penetrates the blood vessels of the ventral epidural space. When peripheral blood has been introduced into the CSF during the performance of the lumbar puncture, a two-step calculation using the peripheral blood and CSF cell count can be performed:

1. a ratio of WBC/mm³:total red blood cells (RBCs)/mm³ is determined for CSF and for peripheral blood; and then
2. a ratio of CSF WBC:RBC to peripheral blood WBC:RBC is determined.

In the presence of bacterial meningitis, the CSF to peripheral blood WBC:RBC ratio is >1, which indicates that the CSF pleocytosis preceded the lumbar puncture procedure.[3] This calculation is based on the assumption that, if the ratio of WBCs to RBCs in the CSF is the same as the ratio of WBCs to RBCs in the patient's blood, then the WBCs were most likely introduced by the spinal tap. If, however, the ratio of WBCs to RBCs in the CSF is higher than the ratio of WBCs to RBCs in the peripheral blood, then the excess of WBCs is due to the presence of WBCs in the CSF prior to the lumbar puncture.[3,4]

An alternate approach is to obtain a WBC count and RBC count on both tube 1 and tube 3. The number of RBCs in the CSF typically decreases between tubes 1 and 3 if a traumatic puncture occurred. Then, if there are >10 WBCs in tube 3, suspect infection. In addition, it is unlikely that a decision on the presence or absence of CNS infection will be based strictly on the number of WBCs in the CSF. The CSF chemistries and Gram's stain are vital to the analysis of the CSF and contribute significantly to the interpretation of the WBC count in CSF.

A CSF pleocytosis has been reported following a flurry of generalized convulsions. The maximum CSF leukocyte count observed was 80 cells/mm^3, and this was obtained 24 hours after cessation of convulsions. It is noteworthy that a CSF pleocytosis may occasionally accompany generalized seizure activity and be secondary to repeated seizures, but should be attributed to seizure activity only as a diagnosis of exclusion.[5-7]

References

1. Conly JM, Ronald AR. Cerebrospinal fluid as a diagnostic body fluid. *Amer J Med* 1983; **75**(1B): 102–6.
2. Dougherty JM, Roth RM. Cerebral spinal fluid. *Emer Med Clin North Amer* 1986; **4:** 281–97.
3. Bonadio WA. The cerebrospinal fluid: physiologic aspects and alterations associated with bacterial meningitis. *Pediatr Infect Dis J* 1992; **11:** 423–32.
4. Mayefsky JH, Roghmann KJ. Determination of leukocytosis in traumatic spinal tap specimens. *Amer J Med* 1987; **82:** 1175–81.
5. Schmidley JM, Simon RP. Postictal pleocytosis. *Ann Neurol* 1981; **9:** 81–4.
6. Lennox WB, Merritt HH. The cerebrospinal fluid in 'essential' epilepsy. *J Neurol Psychopathol* 1936; **17:** 97–106.
7. Petito CK, Shaefer JA, Plum F. Ultrastructural characteristics of the brain and blood–brain barrier in experimental seizures. *Brain Res* 1977; **127:** 251–67.

20.   *The CSF glucose concentration is low when the CSF/blood glucose ratio is <0.6 and/or the value is <40 mg/dL*

The concentration of glucose in the CSF is dependent upon the serum glucose concentration, the facilitated membrane carrier system that transfers glucose between blood and CSF, and the rate of glucose metabolism by the various cellular elements close to the CSF.[1] In purulent CSF, the decreased glucose concentration is due, in part, to increased glycolysis by polymorphonuclear leukocytes in the process of phagocytosis.[1,2]

The CSF glucose concentration is normally lower than that of serum. The normal CSF glucose concentration is between 45 and 80 mg/dL in patients with a serum glucose of 70–120 mg/dL or approximately 65% of the serum glucose. Cerebrospinal fluid glucose concentrations below 40 mg/dL are abnormal. Hyperglycemia increases the CSF glucose concentration and its presence may mask a decreased CSF glucose concentration.[1] The CSF glucose concentration is therefore best determined by the CSF:serum glucose ratio. The normal CSF:serum glucose ratio is 0.6. The CSF glucose concentration is low when the CSF/blood glucose ratio is <0.6. The differential diagnosis of a decreased CSF glucose concentration (hypoglycorrhachia) is:

1. herpes simplex meningoencephalitis;
2. lymphocytic choriomeningitis;
3. mumps meningitis;
4. tuberculous meningitis;
5. fungal meningitis;
6. carcinomatous meningitis;
7. sarcoidosis;
8. hypoglycemia.

A CSF/blood glucose ratio less than or equal to 0.40 is highly predictive of bacterial meningitis. This value has been shown to be 80% sensitive and 98% specific for bacterial meningitis in children older than 2 months of age.[3,4]

The question often arises as to how to interpret the CSF glucose concentration when an ampule of D50 (50 mL of 50% glucose) has been given on arrival in the emergency room. It takes at least 30 minutes, and more likely as long as 4 hours, for the glucose concentration to reach an equilibrium between blood and CSF; therefore, an ampule of D50 will not influence the CSF glucose concentration until at least 30 minutes after it has been given. It should be remembered, however, that in patients who are hypoglycemic, the CSF glucose concentration may be decreased on this basis alone and should be interpreted accordingly.[5]

In preterm and full term infants, the normal CSF/blood glucose ratio is 0.81 due to immaturity of the glucose exchange mechanisms, the greater permeability of the blood–brain barrier to macromolecules, and the much greater rate of cerebral blood flow in infancy compared with adulthood.[1,6]

References

1. Fishman RA. Composition of the cerebrospinal fluid. In: Fishman RA (ed.), *Cerebrospinal Fluid in Diseases of the Nervous System*. Philadelphia: W.B. Saunders, 1992; 183–252.
2. Petersdorf RG, Harter D. The fall in cerebrospinal fluid sugar in meningitis. *Arch Neurol* 1961; **4**: 21–30.
3. Bonadio WA. The cerebrospinal fluid: physiologic aspects and alterations associated with bacterial meningitis. *Pediatr Infect Dis J* 1992; **11**: 423–32.

4. Donald P, Malan C, van der Walt A. Simultaneous determination of cerebrospinal fluid glucose and blood glucose concentrations in the diagnosis of bacterial meningitis. *J Pediatr* 1983; **103:** 413–15.
5. Dagbjartsson A, Ludvigsson P. Bacterial meningitis: diagnosis and initial antibiotic therapy. *Pediatr Clin North Amer* 1987; **34:** 219–30.
6. Conly JM, Ronald AR. Cerebrospinal fluid as a diagnostic body fluid. *Amer J Med* 1983; **75** (1B): 102–6.

21.   *An increased CSF protein concentration is a nonspecific abnormality*

The upper range of normal for the lumbar CSF protein concentration in the adult is 50 mg/dL, and may be as high as 150 mg/dL in the neonate. The higher number for the normal neonatal CSF protein concentration is due to the immaturity of the CSF blood–brain barrier and is therefore a nonspecific abnormality. By 1 year of age, the normal value for the lumbar CSF protein concentration is 45 mg/dL. The normal value for protein concentration in cisternal and ventricular CSF ranges from 13 to 30 mg/dL in adults and from 20 to 170 mg/dL in neonates.[1] An increased CSF protein concentration is typically seen in bacterial meningitis, but the CSF protein concentration will be increased in any process that disrupts the permeability of the blood–brain barrier. When the lumbar puncture has been traumatic, the CSF protein concentration will be increased by 1 mg/dL for each 1000 red blood cells present per mm³.[2]

References

1. Greenlee JE. Approach to diagnosis of meningitis: cerebrospinal fluid evaluation. *Infect Dis Clin North Amer* 1990; **4:** 583–98.
2. Dougherty JM, Roth RM. Cerebral spinal fluid. *Emer Med Clin North Amer* 1986; **4:** 281–97.

22.   *There is typically a predominance of polymorphonuclear cells in CSF in bacterial meningitis, though mononuclear cells may be the predominant cell type or there may be an absence of an increased number of cells in the CSF*

The characteristic CSF abnormalities in bacterial meningitis are as follows:

1. increased opening pressure;
2. polymorphonuclear pleocytosis;

3. decreased glucose concentration (<40 mg/dL and/or CSF/serum glucose ratio of <0.31);
4. elevated protein concentration.

The CSF white blood cell (WBC) count is usually >100 cells/mm³ and is typically markedly elevated with >1000 WBC/mm³. There may be an increase in the CSF total WBC count within 18–36 hours of the initiation of antibiotic therapy.[1,2]

There are reports of bacterial meningitis without an increased number of WBCs in which abnormalities of CSF glucose and protein concentration were the only indicators of infection.[3] In the series described by Fishbein et al.[3], 7 patients with bacterial meningitis had normal CSF WBC counts. All 7 patients were immunosuppressed due to alcoholism, extremes of age (86 years old), or Hodgkin's disease. There was a trend toward higher mortality in the patients with a low initial CSF WBC count. All of the patients had a clinical presentation and a clinical course consistent with meningitis and, in all cases, bacteria were detected in the CSF by Gram's stain or culture. Bacterial meningitis in school-aged children is typically associated with a CSF pleocytosis; however, in premature neonates and in infants younger than 4 weeks of age, bacterial meningitis can be present in the absence of CSF pleocytosis.[4] If the clinical presentation and clinical course are suggestive of bacterial meningitis, the patient should be admitted to the hospital and empiric antibiotic therapy initiated and continued until CSF cultures are negative.

Although bacterial meningitis typically has a predominance of polymorphonuclear cells and viral meningitis typically has a predominance of lymphocytes, there may initially be a predominance of lymphocytes in bacterial meningitis and a predominance of polymorphonuclear leukocytes in enterovirus meningitis with a subsequent shift to a lymphocytic predominance later in the course of the illness.[5,6] It has been suggested that when viral meningitis is suspected and there is initially a predominance of polymorphonuclear leukocytes in the CSF, a repeat lumbar puncture within 6–8 hours will demonstrate a shift to a predominance of mononuclear cells allowing the diagnosis of viral meningitis to be made.[7] This, however, is not always the case. In one series that evaluated the results of a second lumbar puncture 5–8 hours after the initial lumbar puncture in patients with echovirus meningitis, a shift from a polymorphonuclear pleocytosis to a monocytic pleocytosis was not demonstrated.[8]

When a CSF pleocytosis with a predominance of polymorphonuclear leukocytes is obtained, empiric antibiotic therapy for meningitis should be initiated and continued until CSF cultures are negative. A CSF lymphocytosis has been reported in cases of acute bacterial meningitis when the CSF WBC concentration is less than 1000/mm³ and in bacterial meningitis due to *Listeria monocytogenes* .[6,9] A lymphocytic pleocytosis has been reported in 25% of cases of *Listeria* meningitis.[9]

The initial CSF examination in neonatal bacterial meningitis may have an absence of pleocytosis and normal glucose and protein concentrations.[10] A Gram's stain smear of CSF should be examined carefully. A high index of suspicion for meningitis should be maintained in the neonate with fever, seizure activity, irritability, lethargy, and/or respiratory distress, and empiric antibiotic therapy initiated regardless of the findings on examination of the CSF.[11]

References

1. Bonadio, WA. The cerebrospinal fluid: physiologic aspects and alterations associated with bacterial meningitis. *Pediatr Infect Dis J* 1992; **11:** 423–32.
2. Lebel M, McCracken G. Delayed cerebrospinal fluid sterilization and adverse outcome of bacterial meningitis in infants and children. *Pediatrics* 1989; **83:** 161–7.
3. Fishbein DB, Palmer DL, Porter KM, Reed WP. Bacterial meningitis in the absence of CSF pleocytosis. *Arch Intern Med* 1981; **141:** 1369–72.
4. Bonadio WA, Smith D. CBC differential profile in distinguishing etiology of neonatal meningitis. *Pediatr Emerg Care* 1989; **5:** 94–6.
5. Karandanis D, Shulman JA. Recent survey of infectious meningitis in adults: review of laboratory findings in bacterial, tuberculous, and aseptic meningitis. *South Med J* 1976; **69:** 449–57.
6. Powers WJ. Cerebrospinal fluid lymphocytosis in acute bacterial meningitis. *Amer J Med* 1985; **79:** 216–20.
7. Feigin RD, Shackelford PG. Value of repeat lumbar puncture in the differential diagnosis of meningitis. *N Engl J Med* 1973; **289:** 571–4.
8. Harrison SA, Risser WL. Repeat lumbar puncture in the differential diagnosis of meningitis. *Pediatr Infect Dis J* 1988; **7:** 143–5.
9. Cherubin CE, Marr JS, Sierra MF, Becker S. Listeria and gram-negative bacillary meningitis in New York City,1972–1979. *Amer J Med* 1981; **71:** 199–208.
10. Unhanand M, Mustafa MM, McCracken GH, Nelson JD. Gram-negative enteric bacillary meningitis: a twenty-one-year experience. *J Pediatr* 1993; **122:** 15–21.
11. Bonadio WA. Bacterial meningitis in children whose cerebrospinal fluid contains polymorphonuclear leukocytes without pleocytosis. *Clin Pediatr* 1988; **27:** 198–200.

23.   *Oral antimicrobial therapy prior to lumbar puncture will not significantly alter the CSF white blood cell count or glucose concentration*

Antibiotic treatment prior to lumbar puncture may decrease the CSF protein concentration and decrease the likelihood of identifying the organism on Gram's stain smear or isolating the organism in culture, but will not significantly alter the CSF white blood cell (WBC) count or glucose concentration.

It is common for children to have been treated with oral antimicrobial agents prior to a lumbar puncture being performed for the possibility of bacterial meningitis. Both retrospective and prospective studies have determined that initiating antimicrobial therapy prior to CSF analysis is associated with a lower protein concentration and a lower percentage of positive Gram's stain results than in untreated cases.[1-3]

When the appropriate antimicrobial therapy has been initiated for bacterial meningitis, the CSF culture should be sterile and the Gram's stain negative 24 hours after the initiation of therapy. In the majority of patients, the CSF glucose concentration returns to normal within 3 days after therapy is initiated; however, the glucose concentration may remain low for 10 days or longer despite clinical improvement and improvement in CSF WBC count and protein concentrations.[4]

In a review of post-treatment CSF findings in 161 patients cured of bacterial meningitis the following was determined:

1. In 36% of cases, the glucose concentration was below 50 mg/dL; in 8% the post-treatment glucose concentration was below 40 mg/dL.
2. In 38% of cases, the CSF protein concentration was above 45 mg/dL; in 8% the protein concentration was greater than 100 mg/dL.
3. Post-treatment CSF WBC counts were <5/mm^3 in only 28% of cases. The WBC count was $\geq$40/mm^3 in 32% and $\geq$100/mm^3 in 15%.

In this series, there were two infants who were treatment failures and, in both cases, post-treatment lumbar puncture demonstrated normal protein and glucose concentrations and only minimally abnormal cell counts, and therefore failed to predict the presence of ongoing infection.[5] Lumbar puncture should be repeated at the end of treatment only in instances where the clinical condition warrants it.[4,5]

References

1. Davis SD, Hill HR, Feigl P, Arnstein EJ. Partial antibiotic therapy in *Haemophilus influenzae* meningitis: its effect on cerebrospinal fluid abnormalities. *Am J Dis Child* 1975; **129**: 802–7.
2. Kaplan SL, Smith EO, Wills C, Feigin RD. Association between preadmission oral antibiotic therapy and cerebrospinal fluid findings and sequelae caused by *Haemophilus influenzae* type b meningitis. *Pediatr Infect Dis* 1986; **5**: 626–32.
3. Feldman WE. Effect of prior antibiotic therapy on concentrations of bacteria in CSF. *Am J Dis Child* 1978; **132**: 672–4.
4. Fishman RA. CSF findings in diseases of the nervous system. In: Fishman RA (ed.), *Cerebrospinal Fluid in Diseases of the Nervous System*. Philadelphia: W.B. Saunders, 1992; 253–343.
5. Durack DT, Spanos A. End-of-treatment spinal tap in bacterial meningitis. Is it worthwhile? *JAMA* 1982; **248**: 75–8.

24.   Cerebrospinal fluid lactic acid concentration is useful in differentiating bacterial and tuberculous meningitis from aseptic meningitis

An increase in CSF lactate concentrations in bacterial meningitis was first recognized in 1925.[1,2] The CSF lactic acid concentration has been suggested for clinical use as a diagnostic aid in differentiating bacterial and tuberculous meningitis from viral meningitis. A lactic acid concentration of greater than or equal to 35 mg/dL has been suggested to be highly predictive of the presence of meningitis of bacterial or tubercular origin.[3,4]

In one series, all cases of meningitis with CSF lactic acid concentrations >35 mg/dL were of bacterial origin, whereas all cases of aseptic meningitis were associated with CSF lactic acid concentrations <35 mg/dL.[3,5] In another series, CSF lactate concentrations greater than 43 mg/dL were very reliable in differentiating viral meningitis from either bacterial or tuberculous meningitis.[6]

Increased CSF lactic acid concentrations in bacterial meningitis are, in part, the result of anaerobic glycolysis due to diminished cerebral blood flow and brain hypoxia.[2] The CSF lactate concentration is typically elevated in tuberculous meningitis. A CSF lactate concentration ≥39 mg/dL was detected in 21 culture-positive cases of tuberculous meningitis, but the elevated concentration did not correlate with the severity of the illness or the outcome.[7] The CSF lactic acid concentration may not be helpful in cases of partially treated meningitis. The lactic acid concentration declines after treatment of bacterial meningitis; therefore, a low lactic acid concentration should be interpreted cautiously in patients who have been pretreated with antibiotics. In this instance, a high CSF lactic acid concentration is useful; a low CSF lactic acid concentration is not helpful in ruling out the presence of bacterial meningitis. The CSF lactic acid concentration typically remains elevated for weeks despite adequate therapy for tuberculous meningitis.

The CSF lactic acid concentration has a high rate of false positives. The concentration will be elevated in patients who have had previous craniotomies, following closed head injury, in the presence of central nervous system tumors, cerebral ischemia, seizures and subarachnoid hemorrhage.[8-11] Cerebrospinal fluid lactic acid concentrations typically remain elevated for several days post-craniotomy. For this reason it has been suggested that if lactic acid concentrations are to be used in differentiating between bacterial, viral and noninfectious meningitis in neurosurgical patients, the results should be interpreted with caution.[9]

In experimental pneumococcal meningitis, the initial CSF lactate concentration was a strong predictor of survival.[12] The initial CSF lactic acid concentration has also been demonstrated to have prognostic significance in patients with bacterial meningitis. Patients with the highest initial CSF lactic acid levels were more likely to die or recover with a neurologic deficit than those with lower initial CSF lactic acid concentrations.[13]

References

1. Killian JA. Lactic acid of normal and pathological spinal fluids. *Proc Soc Exp Biol Med* 1925; **23:** 255–7.
2. Cameron PD, Boyce JMH, Ansair BM. Cerebrospinal fluid lactate in meningitis and meningococcaemia. *J Infect* 1993; **26:** 245–52.
3. Brook I, Bricknell KS, Overturf GD, Finegold SM. Measurement of lactic acid in cerebrospinal fluid of patients with infections of the central nervous system. *J Infect Dis* 1978; **137:** 384–90.
4. Lauwers S. Lactic acid concentration in cerebrospinal fluid and differential diagnosis of meningitis. *Lancet* 1978; **ii:** 163.
5. Bonadio WA. The cerebrospinal fluid: physiologic aspects and alterations associated with bacterial meningitis. *Pediatr Infect Dis J* 1992; **11:** 423–32.
6. Mandall BK, Dunbar EM, Hooper J, Parker L. How useful is cerebrospinal fluid lactate estimation in differential diagnosis of meningitis? *J Infect* 1983; **6:** 231–7.
7. Tang L-M. Serial lactate determinations in tuberculous meningitis. *Scand J Infect Dis* 1988; **20:** 81–3.
8. Dougherty JM, Roth RM. Cerebral spinal fluid. *Emer Med Clin North Amer* 1986; **4:** 281–97.
9. Lannigan R, MacDonald MA, Marrie TJ, Haldane EV. Evaluation of cerebrospinal fluid lactic acid levels as an aid in differential diagnosis of bacterial and viral meningitis in adults. *J Clin Micro* 1980; **11:** 324–7.
10. Controni G, Rodrigues WJ, Hicks JM, Ficke M, Ross S, Friedman G, Khan W. Cerebrospinal fluid lactic acid levels in meningitis. *Pediatrics* 1977; **91:** 379–84.
11. Simpson H, Habel AH, George EL. Cerebrospinal fluid acid base status and lactate and pyruvate concentrations after convulsions of varied duration and etiology in children. *Arch Dis Child* 1977; **52:** 844–9.
12. Scheld WM, Giampaolo C, Boyd J, Savory J, Wills MR, Sande MA. Cerebrospinal fluid prognostic indices in experimental pneumococcal meningitis. *J Lab Clin Med* 1982; **100:** 218–29.
13. Alam SM, Mitra SK, Vajpeyi GN, Chandra R, Srivastava DR, Sikka KK, Govil MK. Prognostic evaluation of CSF lactic acid in cases of meningitis. *J Indian Med Assoc* 1984; **82**(8)**:** 269–71.

25.   *The CSF C-reactive protein concentration is useful for differentiating bacterial from nonbacterial meningitis in children*

The production of C-reactive protein (CRP) is a nonspecific response to tissue damage.[1] In the presence of CSF pleocytosis, a CSF CRP concentration >100 ng/mL is useful in identifying bacterial meningitis. The CRP has been reported to have a 100% sensitivity and 94% specificity in differentiating bacterial from nonbacterial meningitis in infants (4 weeks and older) and children.[2] The CRP in the CSF of neonates (younger than 4 weeks of age) has not been found to be helpful in differentiating between bacterial and other etiologies of meningitis because the CRP concentration is not consistently elevated in bacterial meningitis in neonates.[3,4]

One of the limitations of using the CRP concentration in CSF to distinguish bacterial from viral meningitis is that the CRP concentration may be low in patients with bacterial meningitis who have a low-grade pleocytosis (<10 white blood cells/μL) due to a minimal inflammatory response. The inflammatory response may be poor or delayed in group B streptococcal sepsis in neonates and young infants, in the early stages of meningococcal infections and with prior antibiotic therapy. In addition, patients who are immunosuppressed may mount a minimal inflammatory response to infection. In all of these cases the CRP in CSF would not be reliable in differentiating between bacterial and viral meningitis.[5]

References

1. Dougherty JM, Roth RM. Cerebral spinal fluid. *Emer Med Clin North Amer* 1986; **4:** 281–97.
2. Corrall CJ, Pebble JM, Moxon ER, et al. C-reactive protein in spinal fluid of children with meningitis. *J Pediatr* 1981; **99:** 365–9.
3. Phillip AGS, Baker CJ. Cerebrospinal fluid C-reactive protein in neonatal meningitis. *J Pediatr* 1983; **102:** 715–17.
4. Dagbjartsson A, Ludvigsson P. Bacterial meningitis: diagnosis and initial antibiotic therapy. *Pediatr Clin North Amer* 1987; **34:** 219–30.
5. Gray BM, Simmons DR, Mason H, Barnum S, Volanakis JE. Quantitative levels of C-reactive protein in cerebrospinal fluid in patients with bacterial meningitis and other conditions. *J Pediatr* 1986; **108:** 665–70.

26.   *Bacterial antigen tests on CSF are useful in making a diagnosis of bacterial meningitis in patients who have been pretreated with antibiotics and in those cases where the Gram's stain and CSF culture are negative*

Several techniques are available to detect bacterial antigens in CSF including the Phadebact coagglutination (CoA) test, the Directigen latex agglutination (LA) test, counterimmunoelectrophoresis (CIE) and the Limulus amebocyte lysate (LAL) test. Today, most hospital laboratories use the latex particle agglutination test for the detection of bacterial antigens in the CSF, and use the LAL test for detection of gram-negative endotoxin in CSF. The LA test has a sensitivity of 78–86% for detection of *Haemophilus influenzae* type b (Hib) in CSF, a sensitivity of 69–100% for detection of *Streptococcus pneumoniae* in CSF and a sensitivity of 33–70% for detection of *Neisseria meningitidis*. The LA test has a specificity of 100% for Hib, 96% for *S. pneumoniae* and 100% for *N. meningitidis*. The LAL assay has a 77–99% sensitivity for the detection of gram-negative endotoxin in CSF.[1–8]

The CoA test is reported to have a sensitivity of 71–83% for detection of Hib bacterial antigens, a sensitivity of 50–71% for *S. pneumoniae* and a sensitivity of 17–100% for detection of *N. meningitidis* in the CSF. The CoA test has a specificity of 97% for Hib and 96% for *S. pneumoniae*. The LA test has a higher sensitivity for the detection of *S. pneumoniae* bacterial antigens than the CoA test. Both the LA and CoA tests are highly sensitive and specific for the detection of *H. influenzae* in CSF; however, the detection of *N. meningitidis* by either of these tests is only about 50% accurate. The LA and CoA tests have replaced the CIE test because they are easier to do and can be done more rapidly than the CIE test.[1,9]

The LAL test is very sensitive in detecting gram-negative bacterial meningitis. The test is reported to have a sensitivity of 99.5% and a specificity of 86–99.8%.[1,10]

Tests for the detection of bacterial antigen are clinically useful in two situations. First, in the patient with a clinical presentation and CSF analysis suggestive of bacterial meningitis but with negative results on Gram's stain, the bacterial antigen test may identify the organism. Second, in the patient who has been pretreated with either parenteral or oral antibiotic therapy. Under these circumstances, the Gram's stain may be negative, but the bacterial antigen test may identify the organism. The interpretation of a positive bacterial antigen test in a child who has recently been immunized against Hib should, however, be interpreted cautiously.[11] A positive CSF antigen test may be due to recent immunization though, in this instance, the CSF white blood cell count and protein and glucose concentrations should be normal.[2,11]

References

1. Hoban DJ, Witwicki E, Hammond GW. Bacterial antigen detection in cerebrospinal fluid of patients with meningitis. *Diagn Microbiol Infect Dis* 1985; **3**: 373–9.
2. Maxson S, Lewno MJ, Schutze GE. Clinical usefulness of cerebrospinal fluid bacterial antigen studies. *J Pediatr* 1994; **125**: 235–8.
3. Bortolussi R, Wort AJ, Casey S. The latex agglutination test versus counterimmunoelectrophoresis for rapid diagnosis of bacterial meningitis. *Can Med Assoc J* 1982; **127**: 489–93.
4. Burans JP, El Tayeb M, Abu-Elyazeed R, Woody JN. Comparison of latex agglutination with established bacteriological tests for diagnosis of cerebrospinal meningitis. *Lancet* 1989; **i**: 158–9.
5. Ballard TL, Roe MH, Wheeler RC, Todd JK, Glode MP. Comparison of three latex agglutination kits and counterimmunoelectrophoresis for the detection of bacterial antigens in a pediatric population. *Pediatr Infect Dis J* 1987; **6**: 630–4.
6. Ingram DL, Pearson AW, Occhiuti AR. Detection of bacterial antigens in body fluids with the Wellcogen *Haemophilus influenzae* b, *Streptococcus pneumoniae*, and *Neisseria meningitidis* (ACYW 135) latex agglutination tests. *J Clin Microbiol* 1983; **18**: 1119–21.
7. Thirumoorthi MC, Dajani AS. Comparison of staphylococcal coagglutination, latex agglutination, and counterimmunoelectrophoresis for bacterial antigen detection. *J Clin Microbiol* 1979; **9**: 28–32.

8. Tilton RC, Dias F, Ryan RW. Comparative evaluation of three commercial products and counterimmunoelectrophoresis for the detection of antigens in cerebrospinal fluid. *J Clin Microbiol* 1984; **20:** 231–4.

9. Kaplan SL. Antigen detection in cerebrospinal fluid – pros and cons. *Amer J Med* 1983; **75** (1B): 109–18.

10. Dwelle TL, Dunkle LM, Blair L. Correlation of cerebrospinal fluid endotoxin-like activity with clinical and laboratory variables in gram-negative bacterial meningitis in children. *J Clin Microbiol* 1987; **25:** 856–8.

11. Darville T, Jacobs RF, Lucas RA, Caldwell B. Detection of *Hemophilus influenzae* type b antigen in cerebrospinal fluid after immunization. *Pediatr Infect Dis J* 1992; **11:** 243–4.

5
Etiologic Organism

27. *Group B streptococci and* Escherichia coli *are the major etiologic organisms of neonatal meningitis*

Neonates

In the first month to 6 weeks of life, group B streptococci and gram-negative bacilli, mainly *Escherichia coli*, account for most cases of bacterial meningitis. Bacterial meningitis in neonates has been divided into two types, early-onset (occurring during the first 7 days of life) and late-onset meningitis (occurring from 8 days to 6 weeks after birth). In early-onset disease, the organism is acquired by the neonate from the maternal genital tract during delivery. Acquisition of this infection is associated with premature and prolonged rupture of amniotic membranes (>18 h) and low birth weight (<2.5 kg). The source of the organism in late-onset disease is presumed to be from other colonized infants or nursery personnel, as 40% of affected infants are born to culture-negative mothers.[1] Group B streptococci are a common cause of both early-onset and late-onset meningitis, whereas *E. coli* more commonly causes early-onset meningitis.[2]

In a review of gram-negative enteric bacillary meningitis in 98 neonates, infants and children (ages 1 day to 2 years), predisposing factors were identified in 25 patients (26%), the most common of which were neural tube defects and urinary tract anomalies. Seventy-three percent were neonates less than 28 days of age at the onset of symptoms. The causative agents were *E. coli* (53%), *Klebsiella–Enterobacter* species (16%), *Citrobacter diversus* (9%), *Salmonella* species (9%) and other gram-negative enteric bacilli.[3]

The neonate is particularly vulnerable to invasive bacterial disease because of inadequate maturation of antibody and cell-mediated immunity, and because the meningeal barrier in neonates offers less protection to meningeal pathogens than in older children and adults.[3,4] *Listeria monocytogenes* is the third most common etiological organism of neonatal meningitis.[5] *L. monocytogenes* is a pathogen in neonates because of a lack of cell-mediated immunity, an important factor in resistance to infection by this organism.[4]

The predisposing factors to neonatal meningitis include:

1. low-birth-weight (<2.5 kg);
2. premature and prolonged rupture of amniotic membranes;
3. aspiration of amniotic fluid;

4. maternal uterine and urinary tract infection;
5. respiratory tract, urinary tract and gastrointestinal tract infections in the neonate;
6. exposure to humidification apparatus, resuscitation equipment and nursery personnel;
7. lack of cell- and antibody-mediated immunity in the neonate.[6]

The clinical presentation of meningitis in the neonate is often subtle. The neonate with meningitis may be either febrile or hypothermic, may manifest the illness with respiratory or feeding abnormalities, and may exhibit neutropenia instead of leukocytosis. Nuchal rigidity and/or a bulging fontanel are not typically found in the neonate, and the first sign of central nervous system infection is lethargy and seizures.[7] Evidence of pneumonia, gastroenteritis or other infection in a neonate increases the possibility of meningitis, and therefore meningitis should be considered in all newborns who are ill.[8]

References

1. Tunkel AR, Scheld WM. Acute meningitis. In: Stein, et al. (eds), *Internal Medicine*. St Louis: Mosby, 1994; 1886–98.
2. Smith AL, Haas J. Neonatal bacterial meningitis. In: Scheld WM, Whitley RJ, Durack DT (eds), *Infections of the Central Nervous System*. New York: Raven Press, 1991; 313–33.
3. Unhanand M, Mustafa MM, McCracken GH, Nelson JD. Gram-negative enteric bacillary meningitis: a twenty-one-year experience. *J Pediatr* 1993; **122:** 15–21.
4. Wenger JD, Hightower AW, Facklam RR, Gaventa S, Broome CV. Bacterial meningitis in the United States, 1986: report of a multistate surveillance study. *J Infect Dis* 1990; **162:** 1316-23.
5. Shattuck KE, Chonmaitree T. The changing spectrum of neonatal meningitis over a fifteen-year period. *Clin Pediatr* 1992; **31**(3): 130–6.
6. Overall JC. Neonatal bacterial meningitis. *J Pediatr* 1970; **76:** 499–511.
7. Bell WE. Bacterial meningitis in children: selected aspects. *Pediatr Clin North Am* 1992; **39:** 651–68.
8. Groover RV, Sutherland JM, Landing BH. Purulent meningitis in newborn infants. *N Engl J Med* 1961; **264:** 1115–21.

28.   *The most common bacterial pathogens of childhood meningitis are* Haemophilus influenzae *and* Neisseria meningitidis

Children

The most common etiological organisms of bacterial meningitis in children are *Haemophilus influenzae* type b (Hib), *Neisseria meningitidis* and *Streptococcus pneumoniae*. Until the vaccination of children with the Hib conjugate vaccines became routine practice, Hib was the most common etiological organism of bacterial meningitis in childhood. The incidence of Hib meningitis has declined dramatically since licensure of the first conjugate Hib vaccine in December 1987 for routine use in children ≥18 months of age, and in October 1990 for use in infants ≥2 months of age.[1]

The characteristic symptoms of bacterial meningitis in children are fever, irritability, altered level of consciousness (lethargy, stupor or coma), vomiting, headache and neck stiffness.[2]

Haemophilus influenzae meningitis

Haemophilus influenzae meningitis is a disease of children between the ages of 6 months and 6 years (most cases occurring in children less than 18 months old), with capsular type b strains accounting for greater than 90% of cases.[3] Host factors that may predispose to meningitis include sickle cell disease, splenectomy, hypogammaglobulinemia and CSF fistula.[4] The presentation of this illness is either that of a subacute infection or an acute fulminant illness. Children with a subacute presentation often have a history of an upper respiratory infection or an otitis media that is followed by fever, lethargy and nuchal rigidity. The fulminant presentation of this illness is characterized by signs and symptoms of meningeal irritation and increased intracranial pressure. Seizures occur in 30–40% of children with *H. influenzae* meningitis and typically develop during the first 3 days of illness.[5] Ataxia may be the presenting sign of bacterial meningitis in a child, especially when the etiologic organism is *H. influenzae*. Focal neurologic signs, such as hemiparesis and cranial nerve palsies, may develop in children with bacterial meningitis either early or late in the course of the illness. Subdural effusions commonly develop in children with *H. influenzae* meningitis and are not typically clinically significant unless they create a mass effect with a subsequent hemiparesis. At least 50% of children with *H. influenzae* meningitis will develop hyponatremia and the syndrome of inappropriate secretion of antidiuretic hormone (SIADH).[6]

Meningococcal meningitis

Meningitis due to *N. meningitidis* is most common in children and young adults. *N. meningitidis* meningitis may occur in epidemics (usually due to serogroups A and C). Congenital (late component) complement deficiencies (C_5, C_6, C_7, C_8 and possibly C_9) are risk factors for meningococcemia.[3] The typical symptoms of meningococcal meningitis are fever, vomiting, lethargy, neck stiffness and headache. The presence of a diffuse erythematous maculopapular rash resembling a viral exanthem may be an early manifestation of meningococcemia, though these lesions rapidly become petechial.[7] Petechiae are found on the trunk and lower extremities (Fig. 28.1), in the mucous membranes and conjunctiva and occasionally on the palms and soles.

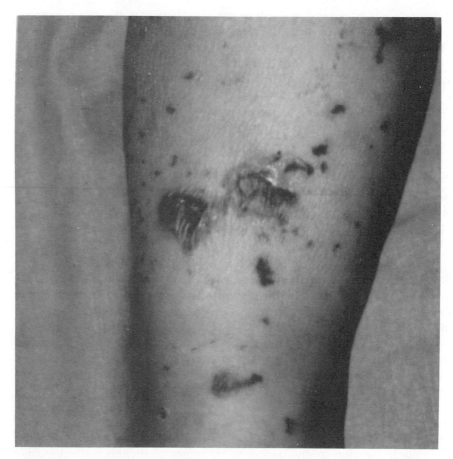

Fig. 28.1   Petechial lesions of meningococcemia.

A few differences in the clinical presentation of *H. influenzae* and *N. meningitidis* meningitis should be emphasized. The presence of a petechial rash is highly suggestive of meningococcemia; however, petechiae are rarely seen in *H. influenzae*, pneumococcal and staphylococcal meningitis. Other infectious diseases that may manifest with a petechial, purpuric or erythematous maculopapular rash like that of meningococcemia are listed in Table 28.1.[8–10] A petechial rash has been reported to occur in 15–62% of cases of meningococcal meningitis.[11–13] Blood obtained from the cutaneous purpuric lesions may reveal the organism on Gram's stain.[8]

The term Waterhouse–Friderichsen syndrome historically has referred to an acute fulminating infectious disease with widespread petechial or purpuric skin lesions, septic shock and death. Bilateral, massive adrenal hemorrhages were the pathologic hallmark sign of this condition. Meningococci were first isolated from the blood of a man who died of adrenal hemorrhage in 1906.[14] Shortly thereafter the meningococcus was recognized as the prime offender in fulminating infectious disease with

Table 28.1 Differential diagnosis of a rash in acute bacterial meningitis

Meningococcemia
Haemophilus influenzae meningitis
Pneumococcal meningitis
Enteroviral meningitis
Rocky Mountain spotted fever
Echovirus type 9
Neisseria gonorrheae sepsis
Staphylococcus aureus endocarditis

purpuric skin lesions and adrenal hemorrhage. Waterhouse and Friderichsen are credited with the description of the syndrome, as each had described a case in 1911 and 1918.[15,16] This fulminating illness was given the label Waterhouse–Friderichsen syndrome in 1933, and by 1943 approximately 107 cases of fulminating infection with adrenal hemorrhage had been recorded.[17] By 1948, the disseminated intravascular coagulopathy that is well known today was recognized as part of this syndrome. The syndrome is characterized by the following:

1. sudden onset of a febrile illness;
2. large petechial hemorrhages in the skin and mucous membranes (Fig. 28.2);
3. septic shock;
4. disseminated intravascular coagulation.

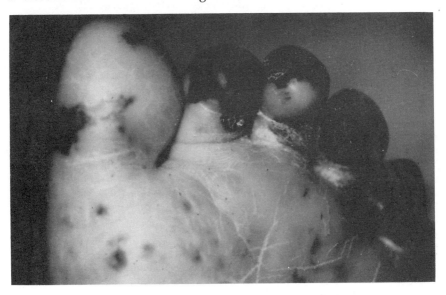

Fig. 28.2 Purpuric lesions of the Waterhouse–Friderichsen syndrome.

This syndrome is attributed to fulminating meningococcal septicemia and is reported in 10–20% of children with meningococcal infection.[18,19]

An altered level of consciousness (stupor and coma) and respiratory symptoms are more common in *H. influenzae* meningitis than in meningococcal meningitis.[2]

Meningococcal meningitis and *H. influenzae* meningitis occur throughout the year, but meningococcal meningitis is most common in the winter months and *H. influenzae* meningitis is most common in winter, spring and fall.

References

1. Schoendorf KC, Adams WG, Kiely JL, Wenger JD. National trends in *Haemophilus influenzae* meningitis mortality and hospitalization among children, 1980 through 1991. *Pediatrics* 1994; **93**: 663–8.
2. Valmari P, Peltola H, Ruuskanen O, Korvenranta H. Childhood bacterial meningitis: initial symptoms and signs related to age, and reasons for consulting a physician. *Eur J Pediatr* 1987; **146**: 515–18.
3. Tunkel AR, Scheld WM. Acute meningitis. In: Stein, et al. (eds), *Internal Medicine*. St Louis: Mosby, 1994; 1886–98.
4. Swartz M. Acute bacterial meningitis. In: Gorbach SL, Bartlett JG, Blacklow NR (eds), *Infectious Diseases*. Philadelphia: W.B. Saunders, 1992; 1160–77.
5. Dodge PR, Swartz MN. Bacterial meningitis – a review of selected aspects II: Special neurologic problems, post-meningitic complications and clinicopathological correlations. *N Engl J Med* 1965; **272**: 954–1010.
6. Kaplan SL, Feigin RD. The syndrome of inappropriate secretion of antidiuretic hormone in children with bacterial meningitis. *J Pediatr* 1978; **92**: 758–61.
7. Weinstein L. Bacterial meningitis. *Med Clin North Amer* 1985; **69**: 219–29.
8. Bell WE, Silber DL. Meningococcal meningitis: past and present concepts. *Military Medicine* 1971; **136**: 601–11.
9. Frothingham TE. Echo virus type 9 associated with three cases simulating meningococcemia. *N Engl J Med* 1958; **259**: 484–5.
10. Durand ML, Calderwood SB, Weber DJ, Miller SI, et al. Acute bacterial meningitis in adults: a review of 493 episodes. *N Engl J Med* 1993; **328**: 21–8.
11. Neal JB, Jackson HW, Appelbaum E. Epidemic meningitis. *JAMA* 1926; **87**: 1992–5.
12. Swartz MD, Dodge PR. Bacterial meningitis – a review of selected aspects. *N Engl J Med* 1965; **272**: 725–31, 779–87, 842–8, 898–902, 954–60, 1003–10.
13. Carpenter RR, Petersdorf RG. The clinical spectrum of bacterial meningitis. *Amer J Med* 1962; **33**: 262–75.
14. Andrewes FW. A case of acute meningococcal septicemia. *Lancet* 1906; **i**: 1172–3.
15. Waterhouse R. A case of suprarenal apoplexy. *Lancet* 1911; **i**: 577–8.
16. Friderichsen C. Nebennierenapoplexie bei kleinen kindern. *Jahrb Kinderheilk* 1918; **87**: 109.
17. Martland HS. Fulminating meningococcic infection with bilateral massive adrenal hemorrhage (the Waterhouse–Friderichsen syndrome). *Arch Pathol* 1944; **37**: 147–58.
18. Fredericks JAM. Meningococcal meningitis. In: Vinken PJ, Bruyn GW, Klawans HL, Harris AA (eds), *Handbook of Clinical Neurology*. Amsterdam: Elsevier, 1988; 21–40.
19. Ferguson JH, Chapman OD. Fulminating meningococcic infections and the so-called Waterhouse Friderichsen syndrome. *Amer J Path* 1948; **24**: 763–82.

29. Streptococcus pneumoniae *is the most common etiologic organism of bacterial meningitis in adults*

The typical clinical presentation of pneumococcal meningitis is that of an upper respiratory tract infection during which a meningeal symptom, such as headache, stiff neck or an altered level of consciousness, develops.[1] Pneumonia is present on admission in 25–50% of adults with pneumococcal meningitis. There are a number of predisposing conditions that increase the risk of pneumococcal meningitis, including:

1. pneumonia,
2. acute and chronic otitis media,
3. sickle cell disease,
4. alcoholism,
5. diabetes,
6. splenectomy,
7. organ transplantation,
8. corticosteroid therapy,
9. hemodialysis,
10. head trauma with basilar skull fracture and cerebrospinal fluid rhinorrhea,
11. congenital or traumatic dural sinus fistula (Table 29.1).[2–5]

Table 29.1   Predisposing conditions for pneumococcal meningitis

Pneumonia (25%)	Splenectomy
Otitis media or mastoiditis (30%)	Hypogammaglobulinemia
Sinusitis (10–15%)	Multiple myeloma
Head trauma	Diabetes
Cerebrospinal fluid fistulae, leak	Organ transplantation
Alcoholism	Hemodialysis
Sickle cell disease	

One of the classic descriptions of bacterial meningitis in adults is that by Carpenter and Petersdorf.[1] This review included 209 cases of bacterial meningitis: 63 were caused by *Streptococcus pneumoniae*, 53 were due to *Neisseria meningitidis*, 35 were due to *Haemophilus influenzae* and 58 were due to other bacterial organisms. The onset of meningitis followed three distinct patterns. Twenty-five percent of patients experienced a rapid onset of headache, confusion, lethargy and altered consciousness seeking hospitalization within the first 24 hours. A second group had more slowly progressive symptoms of meningitis for 1–7 days prior to admission. Many of these patients had symptoms of upper respiratory tract infection. In the remaining group of patients, an infection in the respiratory tract developed 1–3 weeks before the first "meningeal" symptoms appeared. The result of physical examination for signs of meningeal irritation were recorded in 199 cases. Stiff neck, Kernig's sign or Brudzinski's signs were present in 161 patients (81%). A petechial rash was present in 33 out of 53 patients (62%) with meningococcal meningitis. In addition, a rash was present in one patient with pneumococcal meningitis and in one patient with *H. influenzae* meningitis. Importantly, the patients with meningococcal meningitis were most alert, and those with pneumococcal meningitis were most often obtunded. Forty-eight out of 53 patients (91%) with pneumococcal meningitis were stuporous or comatose.[1]

In a more recent review of acute bacterial meningitis in adults aged 16 years of age or older, *S. pneumoniae* was the most common pathogen overall (causing 38% of the 253 cases of community-acquired meningitis). Most patients had an abnormal level of consciousness on presentation; 51% were confused or lethargic, 22% were responsive only to pain, and 6% were unresponsive to all stimuli.[6] Similarly, in a review of 178 cases of community-acquired pneumococcal meningitis, 38% of patients were irritable or lethargic on admission, 29% were delirious or stuporous on admission and 20% were comatose.[2]

Focal neurologic signs and/or seizure activity occur more often in patients with pneumococcal meningitis than in patients with meningitis due to other bacteria.[2] The most common focal neurologic deficits are hemiparesis, gaze preference (due either to a hemispheral lesion or a lesion in the pontine horizontal gaze center) and cranial nerve deficits.[6]

Seizure activity may have either a focal or generalized onset, often occurring within 24 hours of admission. Hemiparesis is either due to cerebral infarction, edema, subdural empyema, or a Todd's paralysis following focal seizure activity. Cranial nerve palsies may involve the third, sixth, seventh or eighth cranial nerves. Cranial nerve palsies develop either due to the presence of a purulent exudate in the arachnoidal sheath surrounding the nerve, due to cavernous sinus thrombosis or as a result of raised intracranial pressure. Papilledema, when present, is evidence of raised intracranial pressure, though there may be raised intracranial pressure in the absence of papilledema.

References

1. Carpenter RR, Petersdorf RG. The clinical spectrum of bacterial meningitis. *Am J Med* 1962; **33**: 262–75.
2. Geiseler PJ, Nelson KE, Levin S, Reddy KT, Moses VK. Community acquired purulent meningitis: a review of 1316 cases during the antibiotic era, 1954–1976. *Rev Infect Dis* 1980; **2**: 725–45.
3. Sokalski SJ, Fliegelman RM. Pneumococcal meningitis. In: Vinken PJ, Bruyn GW, Klawans HL, Harris AA (eds), *Handbook of Clinical Neurology*. Amsterdam: Elsevier, 1988; 41–57.
4. Weinstein L. Bacterial meningitis. *Med Clin North Amer* 1985; **69**: 219–29.
5. Tunkel AR, Scheld WM. Acute meningitis. In: Stein JH, Hutton JJ, O'Rourke RA, et al. (eds),: *Internal Medicine*. St Louis: Mosby, 1994; 1886–98.

6. Durand ML, Calderwood SB, Weber DJ, et al. Acute bacterial meningitis in adults: a review of 493 episodes. *N Engl J Med* 1993; **328:** 21–8.

30.   *The most common etiologic organisms of bacterial meningitis in the older adult (50 years of age and older) are* Streptococcus pneumoniae *and enteric gram-negative bacilli*

In the older adult with bacterial meningitis, *Streptococcus pneumoniae* is likely to be the infecting organism when meningitis is associated with pneumonia or otitis media, and gram-negative bacilli are likely to be the infecting organisms when meningitis is associated with chronic lung disease, sinusitis, a neurosurgical procedure or a chronic urinary tract infection.[1] The most common gram-negative bacilli causing meningitis in the older adult are *Escherichia coli, Klebsiella pneumoniae, Haemophilus influenzae, Pseudomonas* organisms, *Enterobacter* species and *Serratia* species.[2,3]

The typical clinical presentation of bacterial meningitis in the older adult is fever, with temperatures higher than 101°F (38.3°C) and confusion or more severe altered mental status. Meningismus (resistance to passive flexion of the neck) is a common physical finding in the older individual, and may be secondary to meningitis, cervical spondylosis, parkinsonism or paratonic rigidity ("gegenhalten"). In the presence of nuchal rigidity due to meningitis, the neck resists flexion but can usually be passively rotated from side to side. In the presence of rigidity due to cervical spondylosis, parkinsonism and/or paratonic rigidity, lateral rotation, extension and flexion of the neck are all associated with resistance. In a series of 48 patients with bacterial meningitis aged 60 years and older, fever was present in 79%, a change in mental status was present in 69% and meningismus was present in 54%.[1] In one series of 54 patients (aged ⩾50 years) with bacterial meningitis, confusion was present in 12 (92%) of the 13 patients with pneumococcal meningitis and in 7 (78%) of the 9 patients with gram-negative bacillary meningitis. In addition, altered mental status at the time of diagnosis, had prognostic significance. Patients that were obtunded or comatose on admission were more likely to die than patients that were lethargic. Seventeen of the 24 patients (71%) who died had a moderate to severe impairment of mental status at the time of diagnosis.[2]

In older adults with bacterial meningitis, predisposing conditions such as chronic sinusitis/otitis, chronic pulmonary or cardiac disease, chronic urinary tract infections or a chronic debilitated state (i.e. alcoholism, diabetes mellitus, or a hematologic or malignant disease) are present in 50% of patients.[1,4] Pneumonia, either as a co-existent or complicating condition, a focal neurologic deficit, and seizure activity are present more often in the older adult with bacterial meningitis than in the younger adult (age 15–49 years) with bacterial meningitis.[2]

The most likely etiologies of the focal neurologic deficits in the older adult with bacterial meningitis are cerebral ischemia and/or infarction. The older adult is especially at risk for cerebral ischemia during meningitis because of the likelihood of underlying vascular disease. The role of endotoxins and cytokines has been discussed in chapter 2. It is now known that the number of adhesion receptors for monocytes (such as ICAM-1) is increased on carotid arteries in patients with hypertensive disease.[5,6] The interaction of TNF-alpha, interleukin-1 and monocytes results in the conversion of the cerebral endothelium to a procoagulatory state. The subsequent activation of the coagulation system or of complement then leads to thrombosis.[5] With age and/or hypertension there appears to be an increased number of adhesion receptors for monocytes on cerebrovascular endothelial cells with an increased potential for a procoagulatory state in the presence of the inflammatory cytokines associated with bacterial meningitis.

The mortality is higher in the older adult with bacterial meningitis than in the younger adult. Most series report a mortality rate for pneumococcal meningitis in individuals older than 60 years of age of 30–40%.[1,7]

References

1. Rasmussen HH, Sorensen HT, Moller-Petersen J, Mortensen FV, Nielsen B. Bacterial meningitis in elderly patients: clinical picture and course. *Age and Ageing* 1992: **21:** 216–20.
2. Gorse GJ, Thrupp LD, Nudleman KL, Wyle FA, Hawkins B, Cesario TC. Bacterial meningitis in the elderly. *Arch Intern Med* 1984; **144:** 1603–7.
3. Swartz M. Acute bacterial meningitis. In: Gorbach SL, Bartlett JG, Blacklow NR (eds), *Infectious Diseases*. Philadelphia: W.B. Saunders, 1992; 1160–77.
4. Gower DJ, Barrows AA, Kelly DL, Pegram S. Gram-negative bacillary meningitis in the adult: review of 39 cases. *South Med J* 1986; **79:** 1499–502.
5. Hallenbeck JM. The role of cytokines in the tissue damage of stroke. *Neuroscience Forum* 1994; **4:** 1, 5–6, 15.
6. Siren A-L, McCarron RM, Liu Y, et al. Perivascular macrophage signaling of endothelium via cytokines: mechanism by which stroke risk factors operate to increase stroke likelihood. In: Krieglstein J, Oberpichler-Schwenk H (eds), *Pharmacology of Cerebral Ischemia*. Stuttgart: Wissenschaftlich Verlagsgesellschaft mbH, 1992.
7. Wenger JD, Hightower AW, Facklam RR, Gaventa S, Broome CV. Bacterial meningitis in the United States, 1986: report of a multistate surveillance study. *J Infect Dis* 1990; **162:** 1316–23.

31.   *The most common organisms causing meningitis in the neurosurgical patient are staphylococci and gram-negative bacilli*

Staphylococcal meningitis

Staphylococcal meningitis may follow any type of invasive neurosurgical procedure, but most frequently complicates shunting procedures for hydrocephalus. *Staphylococcus aureus* and coagulase-negative staphylococci are the predominant organisms causing infection in patients with CSF shunts. The majority of shunt infections develop within the first 2 months of the surgical procedure, suggesting that bacteria most often enter the shunt system during the performance of the surgical procedure itself.[1-3]

The initial symptoms of shunt infection are nonspecific and include fever, nausea, vomiting and lethargy. Signs of shunt malfunction include enlarging cranial circumference, tense nonpulsatile fontanel and papilledema, and are secondary to progressive hydrocephalus. Meningeal signs are not a common presentation of shunt infections, occurring in less than one third of patients.[3] Cerebrospinal fluid obtained from lumbar puncture may be suggestive, but is often not diagnostic of shunt infection. There is usually only a modest pleocytosis in the CSF, with an average of 75–100 white blood cells/mm^3. Cerebrospinal fluid protein values range from 15–925 mg/dL.[2,4] The procedure of choice for the definitive diagnosis of a shunt infection is aspiration of the shunt reservoir or valve to obtain CSF for examination and culture.[2,3]

Staphylococcal meningitis also complicates the use of subcutaneous Ommaya reservoirs for the administration of intrathecal chemotherapy. These infections are most likely to be the result of the natural colonization of the skin's surface with coagulase-negative staphylococci, and the necessity of puncturing the reservoir twice weekly for many weeks to administer chemotherapy, with frequent potential for breaches in sterile technique.[5]

Parameningeal foci of infection in the neurosurgical patient that are associated with staphylococcal meningitis include:

1. cranial osteomyelitis,
2. subdural empyema,
3. cranial or spinal epidural abscess,
4. fracture of the cranial bones,
5. facial cellulitis.[6,7]

Staphylococci may infect the meninges by hematogenous dissemination from areas outside the CNS. The most common source of staphylococcal septicemia is either a skin infection or endocarditis.[8] Staphylococcal skin infections arise in postoperative wounds, burns and decubitus ulcers. Indwelling intravenous catheters and ateriovenous shunts or fistulae are also sources of *S. aureus* sepsis.

In infants with neural tube defects, *S. aureus* and *Escherichia coli* predominate as the causative organisms of meningitis. In one series of meningomyelocele (249 cases) and meningocele (13 cases) in neonates and infants, there were 33 cases of bacterial meningitis. *Staphylococcus aureus* was responsible for the majority of cases. These patients developed either an ascending infection from the meningomyelocele or developed the infection from the investigation or treatment of the associated hydrocephalus.[9]

Streptococcus pneumoniae is the most common cause of meningitis in the first few days following traumatic head injury. However, as the interval between the head injury and the development of meningitis lengthens beyond 5 days, other organisms, including *S. aureus* and *H. influenzae*, assume increasing predominance among the causative agents. Meningitis develops in the setting of a traumatic head injury in association with the formation of a dural sinus fistula. The most frequent site for a dural sinus fistula is in the area of the cribriform plate. A fracture in this area allows CSF to leak through the arachnoid and dura into the nasal cavity, resulting in CSF rhinorrhea.[10] A small piece of meninges and its vascular connections are trapped in the cribriform plate at the fracture site and allow for the ingress of micro-organisms into the CNS.[6]

Gram-negative bacillary meningitis

The group of patients at risk for gram-negative bacillary meningitis are the elderly, those with chronic and debilitating diseases, such as diabetes, cirrhosis or alcoholism, immunosuppressed patients, infants with neural tube defects and urinary tract anomalies, adults with skull fracture and neurosurgical patients.[11–13] The postsurgical patient with chronic illness (diabetes, alcoholism) or immunosuppression is at greatest risk. The most common neurosurgical procedures resulting in postoperative gram-negative bacillary meningitis are craniotomy for trauma or for tumor.[14] In many cases, gram-negative bacillary meningitis is a nosocomial infection, and this diagnosis should be suspected in patients who develop meningitis during a prolonged hospitalization. The most common gram-negative organisms to cause meningitis in neurosurgical patients are *Klebsiella pneumoniae*, *E. coli*, *Pseudomonas aeruginosa* and *Acinetobacter* species.[14,15] The interval between the neurosurgical procedure and the development of meningitis is often greater than 1 week, suggesting that the infection is most often acquired during the postoperative period rather than at the time of the operation. Local or hematogenous spread of bacteria from distant foci occurs to devitalized tissue at operative sites or to CNS foreign bodies such as indwelling intrathecal or intraventricular catheters. In one review of gram-negative bacillary meningitis in 35 neurosurgical patients, the meningeal pathogen was isolated from another site before or on the same day as the initial isolation of the organism from the CSF in 76% (26 of 34) of the patients.[15] Meningitis may also develop from a contiguous postoperative or traumatic wound infection.[14] In cases of *P. aeruginosa* meningitis in neurosurgical patients, prior colonization of the upper respiratory tract by *P. aeruginosa*, followed by operative or traumatic dural fistula formation between the subarachnoid space and nasal cavities, is thought to play a major role in the pathogenesis of meningitis.[16]

The diagnosis of meningitis in the postoperative patient is most frequently made when lumbar puncture is done for a persistently abnormal mental status. The characteristic signs and symptoms of meningitis (decreased level of consciousness, headache and nuchal rigidity) are so frequently seen in patients that have undergone a neurosurgical procedure that their presentation may be attributed to the surgical procedure itself rather than to the development of infection. The majority of these patients with meningitis, however, will have fever, typically with temperatures above 38°C. In Mangi's review of gram-negative meningitis in 35 neurosurgical patients, temperatures above 38°C were observed in 73% of the neurosurgical patients with meningitis.[15] Because of the difficulty in recognizing meningitis clinically in the neurosurgical patient, a high index of suspicion should be maintained together with a willingness to perform lumbar puncture readily.

References

1. George R, Leibrock L, Epstein M. Long-term analysis of cerebrospinal fluid shunt infections: a 25-year experience. *J Neurosurg* 1979; **51**: 804–11.
2. Forward KR, Ferver HD, Stiver HG. Cerebrospinal fluid shunt infections: a review of 35 infections in 32 patients. *J Neurosurg* 1983; **59**: 389–94.
3. Schoenbaum SC, Gardner P, Shillito J. Infections of cerebrospinal fluid shunts: epidemiology, clinical manifestations, and therapy. *J Infect Dis* 1975; **131**: 543–52.
4. Gardner P, Leipzig T, Phillips P. Infections of central nervous system shunts. *Med Clin North Amer* 1985; **69**(2): 297–314.
5. Trump DL, Grossman SA, Thompson G, Murray K. CSF infections complicating the management of neoplastic meningitis: clinical features and results of therapy. *Arch Intern Med* 1982; **142**: 583–6.
6. Swartz MN, Dodge PR. Bacterial meningitis – a review of selected aspects. *N Engl J Med* 1965; **272**: 725–31, 842–8.
7. Roberts FJ, Smith JA, Wagner KR. Staphylococcus aureus meningitis: 26 years' experience at Vancouver General Hospital. *Can Med Assoc J* 1983; **128**: 1418–20.
8. Hieber JP, Nelson AJ, McCracken GH. Acute disseminated staphylococcal disease in childhood. *Am J Dis Child* 1977; **131**: 181–5.
9. Lorber J, Segall M. Bacterial meningitis in spina bifida cystica: review of 37 cases. *Arch Dis Child* 1962; **37**: 300–8.
10. Hirschman JV. Bacterial meningitis following closed cranial trauma. In: Sande MA, Smith AL, Root RK (eds), *Bacterial meningitis*. New York: Churchill Livingstone, 1985; 95–104.
11. Cherubin CE, Marr JS, Sierra MF, Becker S. Listeria and gram-negative bacillary meningitis in New York City, 1972–1979: frequent causes of meningitis in adults. *Amer J Med* 1981; **71**: 199–209.
12. Mancebo J, Domingo P, Blanch L, Coll P, et al. Post-neurosurgical and spontaneous gram-negative bacillary meningitis in adults. *Scand J Infect Dis* 1986; **18**: 533–8.

13. Unhanand M, Mustafa MM, McCracken GH, Nelson JD. Gram-negative enteric bacillary meningitis: a twenty-one-year experience. *J Pediatr* 1993; **122:** 15–21.
14. Berk SL, McCabe WR. Meningitis caused by gram-negative bacilli. *Ann Intern Med* 1980; **93:** 253–60.
15. Mangi RJ, Quintiliani R, Andriole VT. Gram-negative bacillary meningitis. *Am J Med* 1975; **59:** 829–36.
16. Mombelli G, Klastersky J, Coppens L, Daneau D, Nubourgh Y. Gram-negative bacillary meningitis in neurosurgical patients. *J Neurosurg* 1983; **59:** 634–41.

32. *The etiology of bacterial meningitis in the patient with cancer can be predicted based on the specific type of immune abnormality caused by the cancer or its therapy*

In general, there are three types of immune abnormalities in patients with cancer:

1. a defective neutrophil function or number;
2. a decreased ability to mount an antibody response to a bacterial challenge due to a deficiency in immunoglobulin synthesis and/or splenectomy;
3. a disorder of impaired cell-mediated immunity involving T-lymphocytes and macrophages.

A patient with cancer may have more than one immune abnormality.

The most common cause of opportunistic infections in cancer patients is neutropenia due to either leukemia, or aplastic anemia or pancytopenia due to marrow invasion or intensive chemotherapy or radiotherapy. An increased risk of infection begins with an absolute neutrophil count of <1000 cells/mm^3 and increases as the count drops below 500 cells/mm^3.[1,2] Meningitis in neutropenic patients is usually due to the enteric gram-negative bacilli that reside in the gastrointestinal tract, *Pseudomonas aeruginosa*, *Escherichia coli*, *Klebsiella* and *Enterobacter* species. Of these gram-negative bacilli, *P. aeruginosa* is the most common cause of bacterial meningitis in patients with neutropenia. These patients are also at risk of meningitis due to hematogenous dissemination of *Staphylococcus aureus* and coagulase-negative staphylococci infections of hyperalimentation and other central intravenous lines, or decubitus ulcers from prolonged bedrest (Table 32.1).[1,3]

Patients who are profoundly neutropenic are often also thrombocytopenic, and therefore a platelet count should be obtained prior to the insertion of the lumbar spinal needle for CSF analysis. A platelet count of 50,000 or less should prompt platelet transfusion before lumbar puncture.

Individuals with chronic lymphocytic leukemia, multiple myeloma, Hodgkin's disease and congenital or acquired hypogammaglobulinemia

Table 32.1   Predicting the etiologic organism of bacterial meningitis in the immunosuppressed patient

Type of immune abnormality	Etiology of immune abnormality	Meningeal pathogen
Neutropenia ($<1000/mm^3$)	Chemotherapy Radiotherapy Leukemia Aplastic anemia	*Pseudomonas aeruginosa* *Enterobacter* *Listeria monocytogenes* *Escherichia coli* *Klebsiella pneumoniae* *Staphylococcus aureus* Coagulase-negative staphylococci
Immunoglobulin deficiency	Chronic lymphocytic leukemia Multiple myeloma Splenectomy	*Streptococcus pneumoniae* *Haemophilus influenzae* *Neisseria meningitidis*
T-lymphocyte and macrophage defects	AIDS Organ transplant recipients Lymphomas Adrenocorticosteroid therapy	*Listeria monocytogenes*

Adapted from Pruitt (1991).[1]

have a decreased ability to mount an antibody response to a bacterial challenge and are at risk of meningitis due to the encapsulated bacteria, including *Streptococcus pneumoniae*, *Haemophilus influenzae* type b, and *Neisseria meningitidis*. Patients with splenectomy can develop fulminant sepsis and meningitis due to encapsulated bacteria that can result in death in a matter of a few hours. The spleen has two roles in protecting the host from bacterial invasion:

1. highly efficient phagocytic cells line the splenic sinusoids and have an important role in the filtering of bacteria;
2. the spleen produces IgM opsonizing antibodies.

The combination of an asplenic state and a defect in immunoglobulin production (as occurs in patients with Hodgkin's disease who have had radiotherapy) can be particularly catastrophic.[2] Meningitis caused by any of the encapsulated bacteria can be fulminant.[2,3]

A defect in cell-mediated immunity involving T-lymphocytes and macrophages occurs in patients with acquired immune deficiency syndrome (AIDS), organ transplant recipients, those with lymphomas and lymphocytic leukemias (and as a result of the treatment of these diseases), and in patients receiving immunosuppressive doses of adrenocorticosteroids.[1,4] Individuals with disorders of cell-mediated immunity are at increased risk for *Listeria monocytogenes* meningitis. The presentation of *L. monocytogenes* meningitis tends to be less acute than bacterial meningitis caused by the encapsulated organisms, and the symptoms of fever and headache may extend over 2–10 days.[5] As the majority of systemic *Listeria* infections result in CNS infection in immunocompromised patients, all patients with *Listeria* bacteremia should undergo lumbar puncture. The manifestations of meningitis in the immuno-compromised patient may be mild or absent because of the host's diminished inflammatory response. Therefore, lumbar puncture should be performed in these patients even though the possibility of CNS infection seems low based on clinical symptomatology.

References

1. Pruitt AA. Central nervous system infections in cancer patients. *Neurol Clin* 1991; **9:** 867–88.
2. Rubin RH, Hooper DC. Central nervous system infection in the compromised host. *Med Clin North Amer* 1985; **69:** 281–96.
3. Armstrong D, Wong B. Central nervous system infections in immuno-compromised hosts. *Ann Rev Med* 1982; **33:** 293–308.
4. Armstrong D. Central nervous system infections in the immunocompromised host. *Infection* 1984; **12:** S58–62.
5. Conti DJ, Rubin RH. Infection of the central nervous system in organ transplant recipients. *Neurol Clin* 1988; **6:** 241–60.

6
Therapy of Bacterial Meningitis

33. *A combination of ampicillin and either cefotaxime or an aminoglycoside should be used for empiric antimicrobial therapy of neonatal bacterial meningitis*

The most common etiologic organisms of bacterial meningitis in the neonate are group B streptococcus, gram-negative organisms such as *Escherichia coli*, *Klebsiella pneumoniae* and *Enterobacter* species, and *Listeria monocytogenes*. Until the meningeal pathogen is cultured from the CSF, a combination of ampicillin and either cefotaxime or an aminoglycoside is recommended. When the infecting organism is identified, antimicrobial therapy can be modified to treat the specific organism. For group B streptococcal meningitis, a combination of ampicillin with an aminoglycoside (gentamicin or amikacin) is recommended until the results of susceptibility tests demonstrate that the strain is susceptible to ampicillin. Table 33.1 lists the recommended antibiotic based on the

Table 33.1 Recommended antibiotics for therapy of bacterial meningitis in the neonate

| Organism | Antibiotic Total daily dose (dosing interval) | |
	Neonates (<1week)	Neonates (1–4 weeks)
Group B streptococci	Ampicillin 100–150 mg/kg/day (every 12 h) *plus* Gentamicin 5 mg/kg/day (every 8 h) *or* Amikacin 15 mg/kg/day (every 12 h)	Ampicillin 200 mg/kg/day (every 6 h) *plus* Gentamicin 7.5 mg/kg/day (every 8 h) *or* Amikacin 30 mg/kg/day (every 8 h)
Enteric gram-negative bacilli	Cefotaxime 100 mg/kg/day (every 12 h)	Cefotaxime 150 mg/kg/day (every 8 h)
Listeria monocytogenes Staphylococci	Ampicillin Vancomycin 20–30 mg/kg/day (every 12 h)	Ampicillin Vancomycin 40 mg/kg/day (every 6 h)

Source: McCracken (1992).[4]

infecting organism, and the recommended total daily dose based on the age of the neonate.

It is a common practice to repeat CSF cultures in newborn infants with meningitis every 24–36 hours until sterile to document bacteriologic cure. The rate of bacteriologic response to antimicrobial therapy is delayed in neonates with meningitis caused by gram-negative enteric organisms. In one series, 13 of 22 neonates with meningitis caused by gram-negative bacilli had positive CSF cultures for more than 2 days after the initiation of antimicrobial therapy.[1] Delayed sterilization of the CSF is associated with a higher incidence of seizures, subdural effusion and hemiparesis during hospitalization, and neurologic abnormalities and moderate to profound sensorineural hearing loss at the time of discharge. The repeat CSF culture is, therefore, a useful prognostic indicator in this age group, though persistently positive CSF cultures do not necessarily imply failure of antimicrobial therapy. A repeat examination of the CSF after 24–72 hours of therapy should be considered in neonates with meningitis due to gram-negative enteric bacilli, and when clinical improvement is not satisfactory.[2]

For meningitis due to *L. monocytogenes* or group B streptococci, 14 days of antibiotic therapy is usually satisfactory. For meningitis due to gram-negative enteric bacilli, antibiotic therapy is generally required for a minimum of 3 weeks or for 2 weeks after the first negative CSF culture, whichever is longer. Re-examination and culture of the CSF is recommended at the end of therapy to be certain the infection has been eradicated.[3]

In neonates with meningitis and multiple indwelling catheters, the possibility of meningitis due to coagulase-negative staphylococci should be considered, and treatment with vancomycin is recommended.

Meningitis occurring in infants 4–12 weeks of age requires empiric therapy that is active against the likely pathogens of the neonatal age group as well as those that cause infection in infants and children. Meningitis in this age group may be caused by *Haemophilus influenzae, Neisseria meningitidis, Streptococcus pneumoniae, Listeria*, group B streptococci or enteric gram-negative bacilli. An appropriate regimen for the initial empiric treatment of patients in this age group is ampicillin and either cefotaxime or ceftriaxone.[4]

References

1. McCracken GH Jr. The rate of bacteriologic response to antimicrobial therapy in neonatal meningitis. *Am J Dis Child* 1972; **123**: 547–53.
2. Lebel MH, McCracken GH. Delayed cerebrospinal fluid sterilization and adverse outcome of bacterial meningitis in infants and children. *Pediatrics* 1989; **83**: 161–7.
3. McCracken GH, Sande MA, Lentnek A, Whitley RJ, Scheld WM. Evaluation of new anti-infective drugs for the treatment of acute bacterial meningitis. *Clin Infect Dis* 1992; **15**(suppl 1): S182–88.
4. McCracken GH Jr. Current management of bacterial meningitis in infants and children. *Pediatr Infect Dis J* 1992; **11**: 169–74.

34.   *A third generation cephalosporin, either cefotaxime or ceftriaxone, is recommended for empiric therapy of bacterial meningitis in infants and children*

The most common etiologic organisms of bacterial meningitis in infants and children are *Haemophilus influenzae* type b (Hib), *Neisseria meningitidis* and *Streptococcus pneumoniae*. The third generation cephalosporins, cefotaxime and ceftriaxone, are very effective against these organisms for the most part. If *Listeria monocytogenes* is a possible pathogen, ampicillin must be added to the empiric regimen. If *Staphylococcus aureus* or coagulase-negative staphylococci are possible meningeal pathogens, oxacillin or vancomycin should be added to the empiric regimen. The recommended antibiotics for the treatment of bacterial meningitis in infants and children are listed by organism in Table 34.1. Once the organism has been isolated and susceptibility data are available, the antibiotic regimen should be modified accordingly.

Table 34.1   Recommended antimicrobial therapy of bacterial meningitis in infants and children

Organism	Antibiotic Total daily dose (dosing interval)
Haemophilus influenzae type b (Hib)	Ceftriaxone 100 mg/kg/day intravenously (in divided doses every 12 h) *or* Cefotaxime 225 mg/kg/day intravenously (in divided doses every 6 h)
Neisseria meningitidis	Penicillin G 250,000–400,000 U/kg/day intravenously (in divided doses every 4–6 h) *or* Ampicillin 150–200 mg/kg/day intravenously (in divided doses every 4–6 h)
Streptococcus pneumoniae	Cefotaxime *or* ceftriaxone (doses are the same as for Hib)
Enteric gram-negative bacilli	Ceftriaxone *or* cefotaxime (doses are same as for Hib)
Listeria monocytogenes	Ampicillin 150–200 mg/kg/day intravenously (in divided doses every 4–6 h)
Group B streptococci	Cefotaxime *or* penicillin G *or* ampicillin
Staphylococci	Oxacillin 200–300 mg/kg/day intravenously (in divided doses every 4 h)
Methicillin-resistant staphylococci	Vancomycin 40 mg/kg/day intravenously (in divided doses every 6 h)

Source: Feigin RD, McCracken GH, Klein JO. Diagnosis and management of meningitis. *Pediatr Infect Dis J* 1992; **11**: 785–814.

Pneumococcal strains relatively or completely resistant to penicillin are increasingly recognized; therefore, all CSF isolates of *S. pneumoniae* should be tested for penicillin susceptibility. Meningitis due to these isolates cannot be adequately treated with penicillin.[1] A third generation cephalosporin (i.e. cefotaxime or ceftriaxone) is recommended for relatively penicillin-resistant strains of pneumococci (penicillin minimal inhibitory concentrations (MICs) of 0.1–1.0 µg/mL). For highly resistant strains (MICs $\geqslant$2 µg/mL), vancomycin is recommended. Children with highly penicillin-resistant pneumococcal meningitis (MICs $\geqslant$2.0 µg/mL) are best treated with vancomycin and cefotaxime or ceftriaxone initially, until the MICs of cefotaxime and ceftriaxone for the organism are known. If the MIC of cefotaxime or ceftriaxone for the pneumococci is $\geqslant$1.0 µg/mL, treatment with vancomycin and cefotaxime or ceftriaxone should be continued. If the MICs are $\leqslant$0.5 µg/mL, treatment with cefotaxime or ceftriaxone is probably adequate. Children with inter-mediately penicillin-resistant pneumococcal meningitis (penicillin MICs of 0.1–1.0 µg/mL) who are treated with cefotaxime or ceftriaxone should be observed carefully for treatment failure.[2]

For meningitis caused by Hib, a 7–10 day course of antimicro-bial therapy is recommended. A 7 day course of antimicrobial therapy is adequate for most cases of uncomplicated meningococcal meningitis. For meningitis due to group B streptococci or *L. monocytogenes*, a 10–14 day course of antimicrobial therapy is usually satisfactory. A minimum of 10 days of antibiotic therapy is recommended for pneumococcal meningitis.[3]

The second generation cephalosporin, cefuroxime, is not recommended for treatment of bacterial meningitis in infants and children. Two studies have documented delayed sterilization of CSF cultures associated with hearing loss in patients treated with cefuroxime.[4,5] In a prospective, multi-center study, 106 children with acute bacterial meningitis were randomly assigned to receive either ceftriaxone or cefuroxime. Delayed sterilization of CSF was more frequent among patients treated with cefuroxime (6 cases) than among those given ceftriaxone (1 case). All 7 patients in this study with delayed sterilization of CSF had Hib meningitis. Two of the 6 patients whose CSF cultures remained positive 24 hours after initiation of cefuroxime therapy later had severe bilateral hearing impairment.[5] In another com-parative trial, ceftriaxone also led to a more rapid clinical response when compared with cefuroxime.[4]

The third generation cephalosporins, cefotaxime and ceftriaxone, are both very active against meningeal pathogens. Ceftriaxone has the advantage of a long serum half-life, and can therefore be administered in a once- or twice-daily dose. Cefotaxime can be administered every 8 hours. In a survey of 69 program directors of pediatric infectious disease fellowships in the United States and Canada, the third generation cephalosporins, cefotaxime or ceftriaxone, were the preferred antibiotics for empiric therapy of bacterial meningitis in children 2 months of age or older. Cefuroxime was not selected by any center in the 1992 survey.[6]

For gram-negative enteric meningitis in infants and children, the greatest reported experience is with cefotaxime either alone or combined with an aminoglycoside.[1,7,8] Cefotaxime is only minimally effective or not effective against *L. monocytogenes, Pseudomonas aeruginosa* and enterococci. Ceftazidime is the recommended antibiotic for bacterial meningitis due to *Pseudomonas* species.

References

1. Kaplan SL. New aspects of prevention and therapy of meningitis. *Infect Dis Clin North Amer* 1992; **6**: 197–214.
2. John CC. Treatment failure with use of a third-generation cephalosporin for penicillin-resistant pneumococcal meningitis: case report and review. *Clin Infect Dis* 1994; **18**: 188–93.
3. McCracken GH, Sande MA, Lentnek A, Whitley RJ, Scheld WM. Evaluation of new anti-infective drugs for the treatment of acute bacterial meningitis. *Clin Infect Dis* 1992; **15**(suppl 1): S182–8.
4. Lebel MH, Hoyt MJ, McCracken GH Jr. Comparative efficacy of ceftriaxone and cefuroxime for treatment of bacterial meningitis. *J Pediatr* 1989; **114**: 1049–54.
5. Schaad VB, Suter S, Borradori AG, Pfenninger J, Auckenthaler R, Bernath O, et al. A comparison of ceftriaxone and cefuroxime for the treatment of bacterial meningitis in children. *N Engl J Med* 1990; **322**: 141–7.
6. Klass PE, Klein JO. Therapy of bacterial sepsis, meningitis and otitis media in infants and children: 1992 poll of directors of programs in pediatric infectious diseases. *Pediatr Infect Dis J* 1992; **11**: 702–5.
7. Jacobs RF. Cefotaxime treatment of gram-negative enteric meningitis in infants and children. *Drugs* 1988; **35**(suppl 2): 185.
8. Kaplan SL, Patrick CC. Cefotaxime and aminoglycoside treatment of meningitis caused by gram-negative enteric organisms. *Pediatr Infect Dis J* 1990; **9**: 810.

35.   *In the course of a lifetime, all conscientious physicians will have treated a number of cases of viral meningitis with a short course of antibiotics*

In some cases, the results of initial examination of the CSF do not clearly distinguish between a bacterial and a viral process. The decision may be made to withhold antimicrobial therapy and repeat the CSF examination after 4–6 hours of close observation in the hospital, with the expectation that the repeat examination of CSF will demonstrate a shift to a predominance of lymphocytes if the meningitis is of a viral etiology, or become more indicative of a bacterial process.[1] Any decision to withhold therapy in the setting of meningitis should take the following into account:

1. There are reports of bacterial meningitis without an increased number of white blood cells (WBCs) in which abnormalities of CSF glucose and

protein concentration were the only indicators of infection.[2]

2. In premature neonates and in infants younger than 4 weeks of age, bacterial meningitis can be present in the absence of a CSF pleocytosis.[3]

3. A CSF lymphocytosis has been reported in cases of acute bacterial meningitis when the CSF WBC concentration is <1000 WBCs/mm³, and in bacterial meningitis due to *Listeria monocytogenes*.[4,5]

4. Patients who are immunosuppressed are unable to mount an inflammatory response to bacterial infection. Treatment for bacterial meningitis should be initiated in these patients if the clinical suspicion is strong despite minimal abnormalities on examination of the CSF.

It is recommended that if the clinical presentation and clinical course are suggestive of bacterial meningitis, and the findings on examination of the CSF are unclear (a lymphocytic pleocytosis, <1000 cells/mm³, normal glucose concentration), empiric therapy for bacterial meningitis should be initiated and continued until the cultures are sterile after 72 hours, and the clinical course is indicative of a nonbacterial process.[1]

References

1. Klein JO, Feigin RD, McCracken GH. Report of the task force on diagnosis and management of meningitis. *Pediatrics* 1986; **78:** S959–82.
2. Fishbein DB, Palmer DL, Porter KM, Reed WP. Bacterial meningitis in the absence of CSF pleocytosis. *Arch Intern Med* 1981; **141:** 1369–72.
3. Bonadio WA, Smith D. CBC differential profile in distinguishing etiology of neonatal meningitis. *Pediatr Emerg Care* 1989; **5:** 94.
4. Powers WJ. Cerebrospinal fluid lymphocytosis in acute bacterial meningitis. *Amer J Med* 1985; **79:** 216–20.
5. Cherubin CE, Marr JS, Sierra MF, Becker S. Listeria and gram-negative bacillary meningitis in New York City, 1972–79. *Amer J Med* 1981; **71:** 199–208.

36.   *Careful attention must be given to fluid management in children with acute bacterial meningitis*

The majority of children with bacterial meningitis are hyponatremic with serum sodium concentrations <135 mEq/L at the time of admission. The degree and duration of hyponatremia in children with bacterial meningitis correlates significantly with the complications and neurologic sequelae of this disease.[1] Hyponatremia is due to the syndrome of inappropriate anti-diuretic hormone secretion (SIADH) which results in free water retention and a dilutional hyponatremia. The incidence of this complication in childhood bacterial meningitis in reported series ranges from 28 to 88%.[1–3]

Every child with bacterial meningitis should be evaluated carefully for hyponatremia caused by SIADH. The diagnostic criteria for SIADH are:

1. hyponatremia with hypo-osmolal serum;
2. inappropriately concentrated urine;
3. continued sodium excretion (urinary sodium of >25 mEq/L);
4. absence of renal or endocrine disease.[4]

The primary treatment of SIADH is fluid restriction. The initial rate of intravenous fluid administration has traditionally been limited to approximately one half of normal maintenance requirements or 800–1000 mL/m²/24 h. This practice, however, has recently received renewed attention. Autoregulation of cerebral blood flow is lost in the course of bacterial meningitis so that a decrease in the mean systemic arterial pressure is associated with a decrease in cerebral blood flow (maxim 8). In experimental pneumococcal meningitis, fluid-restricted rabbits had a greater decrease in mean arterial pressure and cerebral blood flow than did euvolemic rabbits,[5] raising the concern that a rigid adherence to fluid restriction in children with acute bacterial meningitis could adversely affect their cerebral perfusion pressure. Until we have a better understanding of how these observations in experimental meningitis relate to meningitis in children, one reasonable approach would be to limit the initial rate of intravenous fluid administration to approximately three-fourths of normal maintenance requirements (or 1000 to 1200 mL/m²/24 h). The intravenous fluid should be a multielectrolyte solution containing between one-fourth and one-half normal saline and potassium at 20–40 mEq/L in 5% dextrose. Body weight, serum sodium concentration and urine specific gravity should be measured at the time of admission and monitored every 6–12 hours. Once the serum sodium concentration increases above 135 mEq/L, the volume of fluids administered can be gradually increased by increments of 200 mL/m²/day at 6–12 hour intervals. In most cases, the rate of intravenous fluid administration will reach maintenance (1500–1700 mL/m²/day) by 36–48 hours after admission. The serum sodium concentration should be monitored for an additional 2–3 days after maintenance fluid administration rates are reached, because occasionally a child will redevelop hyponatremia and again require fluid restriction.[6]

References

1. Kaplan SL, Feigin RD. The syndrome of inappropriate secretion of antidiuretic hormone in children with bacterial meningitis. *J Pediatr* 1978; **92:** 758–61.
2. Laine J, Holmberg C, Anttila M, Peltola H, Perheentupa J. Types of fluid disorder in children with bacterial meningitis. *Acta Pediatr Scand* 1991; **80:** 1031–6.
3. Feigin RD, Dodge PR. Bacterial meningitis: newer concepts of pathophysiology and neurologic sequelae. *Pediatr Clin North Amer* 1976; **23:** 541–56.
4. Diringer MN, Kirsch JR. Disturbances of sodium and osmolality. In: Johnson RT, Griffin JW (eds), *Current Therapy in Neurologic Disease*. St Louis: B.C. Decker, 1993; 347–52.

5. Tureen JH, Tauber MG, Sande MA. Effect of hydration status on cerebral blood flow and cerebrospinal fluid lactic acidosis in rabbits with experimental meningitis. *J Clin Invest* 1992; **89:** 947–53.
6. Kaplan SL, Fishman MA. Supportive therapy for bacterial meningitis. *Pediatr Infect Dis J* 1987; **6:** 670–7.

37. *Seizure activity is an expected complication of bacterial meningitis and should be treated rapidly and aggressively*

Seizure activity develops in approximately 30–40% of children with acute bacterial meningitis and in greater than 30% of adults with pneumococcal meningitis, typically occurring in the first few days of the illness.

During seizure activity, the increased energy demands of discharging neurons quickly exceeds the supply of oxygen and glucose. Seizure activity must be rapidly and aggressively controlled because it can cause ischemic necrosis in the temporal lobe with loss of cortical neurons, and anoxic ischemic changes in the cerebrum in general.[1] Seizure activity that is not aggressively controlled can lead to status epilepticus.

When seizure activity develops, the first step is to maintain the airway, oxygenation and blood pressure. If possible, an oral airway should be inserted and oxygen should be administered by nasal cannula or mask. Systolic blood pressure should be maintained at normal or high-normal levels using vasopressors if necessary. The serum glucose concentration should be determined and, if hypoglycemia is present, glucose should be administered through an indwelling venous catheter. In adults, an initial bolus injection of 50 mL of 50% glucose is recommended. In children a bolus injection of 2 mL/kg of 25% glucose should be administered. Intravenous thiamine, 100 mg, should precede glucose administration in adults.[2] Anticonvulsants should be administered as discussed below.

Benzodiazepines

1. Diazepam
   Adults: 5–10 mg intravenously.
   Children (5 years of age or older): 1 mg every 2–5 minutes up to a maximum of 10 mg.
   Infants and children younger than 5 years of age: 0.2–0.5 mg slowly every 2–5 minutes up to a maximum of 5 mg.[3]
2. Lorazepam
   0.1 mg/kg no faster than 2 mg/min.

Diazepam and lorazepam may cause respiratory depression or

hypotension. A long-acting anticonvulsant agent must be used in addition to the benzodiazepines.

Phenytoin

1. Adults: 18–20 mg/kg
2. Children: 20 mg/kg.

Intravenous phenytoin should not be administered at a rate faster than 50 mg/min in adults or 1 mg/kg/min in children. Phenytoin should be administered through an intravenous line that contains normal saline only, as it is incompatible with glucose-containing solutions. Phenytoin may cause hypotension, and has a depressant effect on cardiac conductivity and automaticity. Therefore, the electrocardiogram and blood pressure should be monitored in all patients during the intravenous infusion of phenytoin.[3] The rate of infusion should be slowed if the QT interval widens or if an arrhythmia or hypotension develops. To minimize these complications, the rate of infusion should be slowed to 25 mg/min in elderly patients. It is necessary to begin maintenance dosing 24 hours after a loading dose of 18–20 mg/kg.[4]

Phenobarbital

If seizure activity continues after a loading dose of 18–20 mg/kg of phenytoin, an additional 5 mg/kg can be given to a maximum dose of 30 mg/kg. If seizure activity continues, endotracheal intubation should be performed and phenobarbital administered. The recommended dose of phenobarbital for adults and children is 20 mg/kg, and this is given at a rate of 100 mg/min. If seizure activity stops before the entire dose is given, the rate of administration can be slowed, but the full dose should be given to avoid recurrence of seizure activity.

Pentobarbital

If phenytoin and phenobarbital fail to control status epilepticus, pentobarbital is given next. Pentobarbital is given in a loading dose of 5 mg/kg. This is followed by an infusion of 0.5–5.0 mg/kg/h either to maintain a burst suppression pattern on the electroencephalogram or to abolish clinical seizure activity, whichever occurs first.[2]

Rectal administration

In cases where intravenous access is impossible, anticonvulsants (diazepam and valproic acid) can be administered rectally. The response to rectally administered anticonvulsants is slow, however, and this route of administration should only be used if the patient is not actively convulsing. The rectal dose of diazepam is 0.5 mg/kg to a maximum of 20 mg. This is then followed by the rectal administration of valproic acid in an initial dose of 20 mg/kg.[2]

References

1. Kaplan SL, Fishman MA. Supportive therapy for bacterial meningitis. *Pediatr Infect Dis J* 1987; **6:** 670–7.
2. Bone RC. Treatment of convulsive status epilepticus: recommendations of the Epilepsy Foundation of America's Working Group on status epilepticus. *JAMA* 1993; **270:** 854–9.
3. Browne TR, Mikati MA. Status epilepticus. In: Ropper AH (ed.), *Neurological and Neurosurgical Intensive Care.* New York: Raven Press. 1993; 383–410.
4. Leppik I. Status epilepticus: the next decade. *Neurology* 1990; **40**(suppl 2): 4–9.

38.   *There does not appear to be an increased risk of epilepsy following aseptic meningitis, but there is a increased risk of epilepsy following bacterial meningitis*

There is a low incidence of epilepsy after aseptic meningitis. There is an increased risk of epilepsy following bacterial meningitis, especially in those individuals who have seizures in the first few days of infection.[1] Partial seizure disorders account for the majority of the seizure disorders.[1,2]

Marks et al.[3] found a significant association between bacterial meningitis in early childhood (before age 4 years) and intractable epilepsy due to mesial temporal sclerosis (MTS). *Haemophilus influenzae* was the most common causative organism of bacterial meningitis in the children that subsequently developed epilepsy. These children had a fairly uncomplicated course during the acute infection, with minimal neurologic sequelae. These investigators concluded that the "time of the CNS insult" in terms of the child's age, was the most critical factor for the subsequent development of intractable epilepsy with MTS. The developing nervous system, specifically the hippocampus and mesial temporal lobe structures are more susceptible to a variety of insults, compared with the adult nervous system. In uncomplicated meningitis, possibilities for hippocampal damage include direct injury from the infective process itself, high fevers or recurrent seizures.[3]

Children with persistent neurologic deficits due to bacterial meningitis, such as hemiparesis, quadriparesis or sensorineural hearing loss, are at an increased risk of developing epilepsy. In most cases, epilepsy that follows meningitis occurs within 5 years of the acute illness. The cerebral injury during bacterial meningitis that has the highest association with the subsequent development of a seizure disorder is cerebral ischemia.[4]

As early as 1876, John Hughlings Jackson[5] recognized an association between cerebrovascular disease and seizure activity when he wrote: "It is not uncommon to find when a patient has recovered or is recovering from hemiplegia, that he is attacked by convulsion beginning in some part of the paralyzed region, almost always, I believe, the face or the hand".

Richardson and Dodge[6] reviewed the autopsy records of the neuropathology laboratory of the Massachusetts General Hospital to determine the incidence and nature of seizures in association with cerebral hemorrhage and/or infarction. One hundred and four cases of cerebral infarction and/or hemorrhage were selected for review. At least one convulsive seizure occurred in 13 (12.5%) of the 104 cases. Recurrent seizures occurred in 6 (5.8%) of the 104 cases. Gross lesions of the cerebral cortex were found in 57 of the 104 cases. Convulsive seizures occurred in 22.8% of the 57 cases of cortical lesions.[6] Although there are certainly other precipitants to seizure activity in the course of bacterial meningitis, such as hyponatremia, fever and subdural effusion with mass effect, cerebral ischemia with infarction or hemorrhage is clearly important in the pathogenesis of epilepsy during and following bacterial meningitis.

References

1. Annegers JF, Hauser WA, Beghi E, Nicolosi A, Kurland LT. The risk of unprovoked seizures after encephalitis and meningitis. *Neurology* 1988; **38:** 1407–10.
2. Rosman NP, Peterson DG, Kaye EM, Coulton T. Seizures in bacterial meningitis: prevalence, patterns, pathogenesis, and prognosis. *Pediatr Neurol* 1985; **1:** 278–85.
3. Marks DA, Kim J, Spencer DD, Spencer SS. Characteristics of intractable seizures following meningitis and encephalitis. *Neurology* 1992; **42:** 1513–18.
4. Pomeroy SL, Holmes SJ, Dodge PR, Feigin RD. Seizures and other neurologic sequelae of bacterial meningitis in children. *N Engl J Med* 1990; **323:** 1651–7.
5. Jackson JH. In: Taylor J (ed.), Selected writings of John Hughlings Jackson. *Volume I: On Epilepsy and Epileptiform Convulsions.* London: Hodder and Stoughton, 1931.
6. Richardson EP, Dodge PR. Epilepsy in cerebral vascular disease. *Epilepsia* 1954; **3:** 49–71.

39.   *Subdural effusions commonly develop in the course of bacterial meningitis in children, and are typically not associated with clinical symptomatology*

McKay et al. were the first to report the occurrence of subdural effusions in children with bacterial meningitis due to *Haemophilus influenzae* type b.[1,2]

Subdural effusions develop in the course of bacterial meningitis when the infection in the adjacent subarachnoid space leads to an increase in the permeability of the thin-walled capillaries and veins in the inner layer of the dura. The result is leakage of albumin-rich fluid into the subdural space. This is usually a self-limited process and, as the inflammatory process subsides, fluid formation ceases and the fluid in the subdural space is resorbed.[3,4] Surgical drainage of an uncomplicated subdural effusion is usually not indicated.

Some subdural effusions are clinically significant. The indications for aspiration of a subdural fluid collection include a clinical suspicion that the fluid is infected, a rapidly enlarging head circumference in a child without hydrocephalus, focal neurologic findings, and/or evidence of increased intracranial pressure. The presence of a prolonged fever in a child with a subdural effusion may be an indication that the subdural effusion has become infected – a subdural empyema. The latter is best managed by drainage and antimicrobial therapy.[3] A subdural effusion can be distinguished from a subdural empyema by a neuroimaging procedure. On computed tomography scan subdural fluid collections are isointense with CSF whereas a subdural empyema is typically slightly more dense than normal CSF. On magnetic resonance imaging, subdural effusions are isointense with CSF on all pulse sequences whereas the signal intensity of a subdural empyema is higher than that of normal CSF on all pulse sequences.[5]

References

1. McKay RJ, Morissette RA, Ingraham FD, et al. Collections of subdural fluid complicating meningitis due to *Haemophilus influenzae*, type b: a preliminary report. *N Engl J Med* 1950; **242**: 20–1.
2. McKay RJ, Ingraham FD, Matson DD. Subdural fluid complicating bacterial meningitis. *JAMA* 1953; **152**: 387–91.
3. Klein JO, Feigin RD, McCracken GH. Report of the task force on diagnosis and management of meningitis. *Pediatrics* 1986; **78**: S959–82.
4. Dodge PR, Swartz MN. Bacterial meningitis: a review of selected aspects: II. Special neurologic problems, postmeningitic complications and clinico-pathologic correlations. *N Engl J Med* 1965; **272**: 1003–10.
5. Smith RR, Arvin MC. Neuroradiology of intracranial infection. *Semin Neurol* 1992; **12**: 248–62.

40.   *Cranial nerve abnormalities that develop in the course of acute bacterial meningitis usually involve the third, sixth, seventh and eighth nerves, and typically resolve after recovery from meningitis, with the exception of eighth nerve deafness*

The most likely etiology of cranial nerve abnormalities that develop during acute bacterial meningitis is the presence of an inflammatory exudate in the arachnoidal sheath enveloping the cranial nerve (Fig. 40.1). Sensorineural hearing loss is the most common serious complication of bacterial meningitis in infants and children and is more frequent with pneumococcal meningitis than with meningitis due to either *Neisseria meningitidis* or *Haemophilus influenzae*. In a prospective 5-year study of the occurrence and persistence of hearing loss among 185 infants and children with acute bacterial meningitis, the overall incidence of a transient conductive hearing loss (associated with a unilateral or bilateral otitis media) was 16%, and of a persistent unilateral or bilateral sensorineural hearing loss was 10%. Patients with pneumococcal meningitis had the highest incidence of sensorineural hearing loss (31%), followed by *N. meningitidis* (10.5%) and *H. influenzae* (6%). In all the patients in this series, sensorineural deafness was permanent.[1]

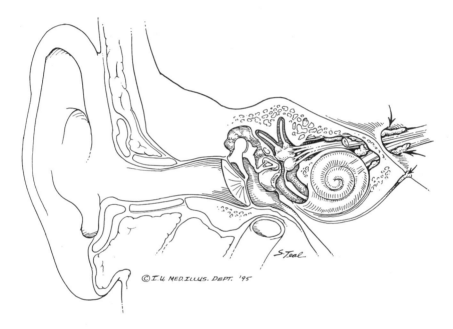

Fig. 40.1   One of the pathogenic mechanisms of sensorineural hearing loss in bacterial meningitis is the presense of an inflammatory exudate (black arrows) in the arachnoidal sheath of cranial nerve VIII.

In a meta-analysis of 45 reports of the outcome of bacterial meningitis published since 1955 involving a total of 4,920 children, the mean probability of deafness was 10.5%, and that of bilateral severe or profound deafness was 5.1%. Deafness was defined as a hearing loss of ⩾30 decibels in one or both ears or classification as hearing loss or deafness by the authors. Children were included in the severe/profound deafness category only if they had bilateral severe or profound hearing loss as defined by the authors. Most studies did not report the specific audiological criteria for these groups, but those that did generally defined severe deafness as a hearing loss of ⩾70 decibels.[2] Approximately 37% of all hearing deficits acquired postnatally are due to bacterial meningitis.[3,4]

One or a combination of the following pathogenetic mechanisms is responsible for sensorineural hearing loss during bacterial meningitis:

1. cochlear dysfunction due to a direct invasion of bacteria into the cochlea via the cochlear aqueduct;
2. cochlear nerve inflammation secondary to the inflammatory exudate in the arachnoidal sheath of the nerve;
3. vascular occlusion of the internal auditory artery;
4. cochlear or nerve toxicity due to antimicrobial agents such as the aminoglycosides or vancomycin.

The pathologic basis of hearing loss was investigated in an animal model of *Streptococcus suis* meningitis. Hearing was evaluated by brainstem auditory evoked potentials. Fifteen of 17 animals with *S. suis* meningitis showed evidence of hearing loss which, on histologic examination, was found to be associated with suppurative labyrinthitis. The 2 animals that did not have hearing loss had normal cochleas.[5]

It is most likely that hearing loss occurs early in the course of infection. Vienny et al.[6] tested hearing within 48 hours of admission and found that patients whose tests were normal did not develop sensorineural hearing loss at a later time, whereas all those who had evidence of persistent sensorineural hearing loss at follow-up had had abnormal test results within the first 48 hours following admission. Dodge et al.[1] found a significant correlation ($P < 0.01$) between sensorineural deafness and initial CSF glucose concentrations of less than 20 mg/dL. No other differences between hearing loss and CSF findings at admission (protein concentrations >200 mg/dL, number of leukocytes >2000/mm^3) were statistically significant.[1]

Seven of 8 children with post-meningitis ataxia had severe to profound sensorineural hearing loss.[7] Ataxia is an uncommon complication of bacterial meningitis, being reported in approximately 3% of children in large series.[7,8] The pathophysiology of ataxia in this infection is most likely the result of labyrinthine dysfunction. The association of ataxia and sensorineural hearing loss suggests involvement of both the vestibular and cochlear divisions of the eighth nerve. Alternatively, there is simultaneous cochlear and labyrinthine dysfunction due to inflammation.

Hearing loss may improve with time. Children who develop hearing loss during the course of bacterial meningitis need close follow-up to detect persistent deficits. The use of corticosteroids as adjunctive therapy to prevent sensorineural hearing loss is discussed in maxim 46.

The basis for the other cranial nerve abnormalities that develop in the course of bacterial meningitis is probably the presence of an inflammatory exudate in the arachnoidal sheath of the nerve causing a compressive and/or inflammatory neuropathy as the nerve courses through its bony canal, or a compressive neuropathy due to increased intracranial pressure.

References

1. Dodge PR, Davis H, Feigin RD, et al. Prospective evaluation of hearing impairment as a sequela of acute bacterial meningitis. *N Engl J Med* 1984; **311**: 869–74.
2. Baraff LJ, Lee SI, Schriger DL. Outcomes of bacterial meningitis in children: a meta-analysis. *Pediatr Infect Dis J* 1993; **12**: 389–94.
3. Smith AL. Neurologic sequelae of meningitis. *N Engl J Med* 1988; **319**: 1012–13.
4. Schildroth AN. Annual survey of hearing impaired children and youth, 1980–1981. Washington, DC: The Gallaudet Research Institute, Center for Assessment and Demographic Studies, Gallaudet College, 1982.
5. Kay R. The site of the lesion causing hearing loss in bacterial meningitis: a study of experimental streptococcal meningitis in guinea-pigs. *Neuropathol Appl Neurobiol* 1991; **17**: 485–93.
6. Vienny H, Despland PA, Lutschg J, et al. Early diagnosis and evolution of deafness in childhood bacterial meningitis: a study using brainstem auditory evoked potentials. *Pediatrics* 1984; **73**: 579–86.
7. Kaplan SL, Goddard J, Van Kleeck MV, et al. Ataxia and deafness in children due to bacterial meningitis. *Pediatrics* 1981; **68**: 8–12.
8. Feigin RD, Stechenberg BW, Chang MJ, et al. Prospective evaluation of treatment of *Hemophilus influenzae* meningitis. *J Pediatr* 1976; **88**: 542–8.

41. *Empiric therapy of community-acquired bacterial meningitis in adults should include either penicillin G, ampicillin or a third-generation cephalosporin*

The most common causative organisms of community-acquired bacterial meningitis in the adult are *Streptococcus pneumoniae* and *Neisseria meningitidis*. Penicillin G, ampicillin and the third-generation cephalosporins, cefotaxime and ceftriaxone, are equally effective therapy for meningitis due to either of these organisms. Experimental studies have shown that the best clinical response is achieved with CSF antibiotic concentrations that exceed the minimal bactericidal concentration (MBC) of the meningeal pathogen by 10–20-fold. Once the infecting organism has been identified and its susceptibilities determined, therapy can be altered accordingly. Table 41.1 gives the recommended antibiotic for the treatment of bacterial meningitis in adults by infecting organisms.

There are an increasing number of *S. pneumoniae* strains that are relatively or completely resistant to penicillin, and some that are resistant to third-generation cephalosporins.[1,2] Penicillin-resistant pneumococcal meningitis is a much greater problem than cephalosporin-resistant pneumococcal meningitis. All of the cases of cephalosporin failure to date have been in children, and the pneumococcus was also resistant to penicillin.[3] A third-generation cephalosporin (cefotaxime or ceftriaxone) is recommended for relatively penicillin-resistant pneumococcal meningitis (minimal inhibitory concentration (MIC) of 0.1–1.0 µg/mL). For highly penicillin-resistant pneumococcal meningitis (MIC ≥ 2.0 μg/mL) vancomycin (with or without the addition of rifampin) is the antibiotic of choice. There are, however, a few reports documenting failure of vancomycin in CSF-culture-proven pneumococcal meningitis, indicating the need for careful monitoring of these patients as well.[4]

Table 41.1   Recommended antimicrobial therapy of bacterial meningitis in adults

Organism	Antibiotic Total daily dose (dosing interval)
Neisseria meningitidis	Penicillin G 20–24 million U/day intravenously (divided doses every 4 h) *or* Ampicillin 12 g/day intravenously (every 4 h)
Streptococcus pneumoniae	Ceftriaxone *or* cefotaxime *plus* vancomycin
Gram-negative bacilli (except *Pseudomonas aeruginosa*)	Ceftriaxone 2–4 g/day intravenously (every 12 h) *or* Cefotaxime 8 g/day intravenously (every 4 h)
Pseudomonas aeruginosa	Ceftazidime 6 g/day intravenously (every 8 h)
Haemophilus influenzae type b	Ceftriaxone *or* cefotaxime
Staphylococcus aureus (methicillin-sensitive)	Oxacillin 9–12 g/day intravenously (every 4 h)
Staphylococcus aureus (methicillin-resistant)	Vancomycin 2 g/day intravenously (every 6 h)
Listeria monocytogenes	Ampicillin 12 g/day intravenously (every 4 h)
Enterobacteriaceae	Third-generation cephalosporin

Source: Roos KL, Tunkel AR, Scheld WM. Acute bacterial meningitis in children and adults. In: Scheld WM, Whitley RJ, Durack DT (eds). *Infections of the Central Nervous System.* New York: Raven Press, 1991; 335–409.

Penicillin or ampicillin remain the antibiotics of choice for treatment of meningococcal meningitis. Strains with relative resistance to penicillin (MIC 0.1–0.7 μg/mL) due to reduced affinity for penicillin-binding protein 3 have been reported. However, conventional therapy with penicillin has been successful in treating most patients infected with these strains.[5]

For the treatment of community-acquired meningitis in adults due to *Haemophilus influenzae* type b (Hib) or Enterobacteriaceae, cefotaxime or ceftriaxone is preferred. *Staphylococcus aureus* meningitis should be treated with intravenous oxacillin. Methicillin-resistant *S. aureus* meningitis should be treated with vancomycin, and vancomycin is the drug of choice for meningitis due to coagulase-negative staphylococci.

Meningitis due to gram-negative bacilli is treated with either ceftriaxone or cefotaxime, except if the organism is *Pseudomonas aeruginosa*. Meningitis due to this organism should be treated with ceftazidime plus a parenteral aminoglycoside for the first week of therapy. Ceftazidime has excellent bactericidal activity against *P. aeruginosa in vitro*. Ceftazidime has good penetration into CSF and peak and trough concentrations are usually several times the MIC against most *P. aeruginosa* strains. The quinolones have excellent activity against gram-negative bacilli *in vitro* and penetrate well into CSF. Despite this, the actual CSF concentration of the currently available quinolones after systemic administration often does not exceed the MIC of these agents against *P. aeruginosa in vitro*. The addition of a quinolone (ciprofloxacin, ofloxacin or pefloxacin) to ceftazidime and/or an aminoglycoside may be beneficial in the treatment of meningitis due to multiresistant strains of *P. aeruginosa*.

Imipenem/cilastatin is not recommended for the treatment of bacterial meningitis due to the standard pathogens as there is a high incidence of seizure activity associated with the use of this antimicrobial agent in dosages indicated for meningitis.[6,7]

Pneumococcal meningitis is treated for 10–14 days, Hib meningitis for 10 days, meningococcal meningitis for 7 days and meningitis due to gram-negative enteric bacilli for 21 days.

References

1. Bradley JS, Connor JD. Ceftriaxone failure in meningitis caused by *Streptococcus pneumoniae* with reduced susceptibility to beta-lactam antibiotics. *Pediatr Infect Dis J* 1991; **10**: 871–3.
2. Sloas MM, Barrett FF, Chesney PJ, et al. Cephalosporin treatment failure in penicillin- and cephalosporin-resistant *Streptococcus pneumoniae* meningitis. *Pediatr Infect Dis J* 1992; **11**: 662–6.
3. John CC. Treatment failure with use of a third-generation cephalosporin for penicillin-resistant pneumococcal meningitis: case report and review. *Clin Infect Dis* 1994; **18**: 188–93.
4. Tunkel AR, Scheld WM. Acute meningitis. In: Stein JH (ed.), *Internal Medicine*, 4th edn. St Louis: Mosby 1994; 1886–99.
5. Swartz M. Acute bacterial meningitis. In: Gorbach SL, Bartlett JG, Blacklow NR (eds), *Infectious Diseases*. Philadelphia: W.B. Saunders, 1992; 1160–77.
6. Kaplan SL. New aspects of prevention and therapy of meningitis. *Infect Dis Clin North Amer* 1992; **6**: 197–214.
7. Calandra GB, Brown KR, Grad LC, et al. Review of adverse experiences and tolerability in the first 2516 patients treated with imipenem/cilastatin. *Am J Med* 1985; **78**(Suppl 6A): 73.

42.   *Empiric therapy of bacterial meningitis in the older adult (50 years of age and older) should include a combination of a third-generation cephalosporin, either ceftriaxone or cefotaxime, with ampicillin*

The most common causative organisms of bacterial meningitis in the older adult are *Streptococcus pneumoniae* and gram-negative bacilli. The specific organism can often be predicted based on the underlying condition or predisposing factors. Fifty percent of cases of meningitis due to *S. pneumoniae* in this age group are associated with pneumonia or otitis media.[1-3] Gram-negative bacilli are likely to be the infecting organisms when meningitis is associated with chronic lung disease, sinusitis or a chronic urinary tract infection.[1] Ampicillin is added to the empiric regimen to cover for *Listeria monocytogenes*. The presence of immunosuppression or chronic disease would favor the addition of ampicillin to the regimen, since *L. monocytogenes* is not susceptible to the third-generation cephalosporins.

Table 41.1 (see maxim 41) lists the recommended antibiotic for the treatment of bacterial meningitis in adults by specific organism. Susceptibility testing on CSF isolates should be performed as discussed in maxim 41.

References

1. Rasmussen HH, Sorensen HT, Moller-Peterson J, Mortensen FV, Nielsen B. Bacterial meningitis in elderly patients: clinical picture and course. *Age and Ageing* 1992; **21:** 216–20.
2. Behrman RE, Meyers BR, Mendelson MH, Sacks HS, Hirschman SZ. Central nervous system infections in the elderly. *Arch Intern Med* 1989; **149:** 1596–9.
3. Carpenter RR, Petersdorf RG. The clinical spectrum of bacterial meningitis. *Am J Med* 1962; **33:** 262–75.

43.   *Acute ischemic stroke during bacterial meningitis is managed in the same way as acute ischemic stroke due to any other etiology*

Acute ischemic stroke that occurs during bacterial meningitis may manifest itself as a focal neurologic deficit, an altered level of consciousness, or with clinical signs of increased intracranial pressure and/or herniation. The etiology of acute ischemic stroke in the course of bacterial meningitis may be one or more of the following:

1. Narrowing of large arteries at the base of the brain. This most often occurs at the supraclinoid portion of the internal carotid artery. The arterial

narrowing is considered to be caused by several mechanisms, either alone or in combination, including encroachment by the inflammatory subarachnoid purulent exudate, infiltration of the arterial wall by inflammatory cells (vasculitis) with thickening of blood vessel walls, and/or vasospasm.
2. Narrowing of medium sized arteries and thrombotic or stenotic occlusion of branches of the middle cerebral artery.
3. Focal hyperperfusion due to dilatation of arterioles and capillaries and premature venous filling.
4. Septic venous sinus thrombosis and thrombophlebitis of cortical veins.[1-5]

An emergency noncontrast cranial computed tomography (CT) scan should be obtained for any patient who appears clinically to have developed a cerebrovascular complication during bacterial meningitis. The risk of an acute ischemic stroke is greatest during the first 5 days of the infection.[2] The CT scan is obtained to rule out an intracranial hemorrhage. The major neurologic complications of acute ischemic stroke, in addition to a neurologic deficit, are increased intracranial pressure due to cerebral edema and seizures after large cortical infarctions. The major medical complications of acute ischemic stroke are aspiration pneumonia, pulmonary embolism, deep vein thrombosis, urinary tract infection and skin breakdown.

To prevent aspiration pneumonia, the head of the bed should remain elevated 30–45 degrees. Impaired swallowing function or an altered level of consciousness may be complications of acute ischemic stroke that prevent oral feeding. Enteral nutrition is the preferred route, but should not be started for the first 24 hours after acute ischemic stroke to prevent aspiration pneumonia from delayed emptying. When enteral nutrition is begun, a nasogastric tube is adequate for the short-term, and gastric residual should be checked every 4 hours. For prophylaxis of deep vein thrombosis, low-dose heparin (5000 IU) should be given subcutaneously every 12 hours. The use of elastic compression stockings and intermittent pneumatic compression has also been shown to decrease the incidence of deep vein thrombosis. Intermittent catheterization is preferable to an indwelling catheter in patients with voiding problems, to prevent urinary tract infections. To prevent decubiti, frequent turning of patients is necessary, and the skin should be kept dry. Blood pressure should be controlled conservatively and not treated unless the systolic or diastolic blood pressure is at or above 220 mmHg or 120 mmHg, respectively.[6]

The use of anticoagulation is controversial as initial management. Haring et al.[2] observed a beneficial effect of heparin therapy in 41 patients with cerebrovascular complications of bacterial meningitis. If heparinization is employed, precautionary measures must be used. Anticoagulation with heparin therapy can cause thrombocytopenia and/or intravascular coagulation from heparin-induced reduction of antithrombin III activity. Platelet count and antithrombin III measurements should be monitored. There is a risk of intracranial hemorrhage with heparin therapy so any worsening in symptomatology should be evaluated with a cranial CT scan.[7] Dose-adjusted intravenous heparin therapy has been reported to be advantageous in patients with aseptic sinus venous thrombosis,[8] but the role of heparinization in the treatment of septic sinus venous thrombosis in bacterial meningitis is not known.

References

1. Pfister HW, Borasio GD, Dirnagl U, Bauer M, Einhaupl KM. Cerebrovascular complications of bacterial meningitis in adults. *Neurology* 1992; **42:** 1497–1504.
2. Haring HP, Rotzer HK, Reindl H, et al. Time course of cerebral blood flow velocity in central nervous system infections: a transcranial Doppler sonography study. *Arch Neurol* 1993; **50:** 98–101.
3. Gado M, Axley J, Appleton B, Prensky AL. Angiography in the acute and posttreatment phases of *Haemophilus influenzae* meningitis. *Radiology* 1974; **110:** 439–44.
4. Igarashi M, Gilmartin RC, Gerald B, Wilburn F, Jabbour JT. Cerebral arteritis and bacterial meningitis. *Arch Neurol* 1984; **41:** 531–5.
5. Lyons EL, Leeds NE. The angiographic demonstration of arterial vascular disease in purulent meningitis. *Radiology* 1967; **88:** 935–8.
6. Adams RJ. Management issues for patients with ischemic stroke. *Neurology* 1995; **45**(Suppl 1): S15–18.
7. Haring HP, Berek K, Kampfl A. Letters to the Editor. *Arch Neurol* 1994; **50:** 98.
8. Einhaupl KM, Villringer A, Meister W, et al. Heparin treatment in sinus venous thrombosis. *Lancet* 1991; **338:** 597–600.

44.   Empiric antimicrobial therapy of bacterial meningitis in the neurosurgical patient should include a combination of a third-generation cephalosporin, plus oxacillin or vancomycin, and an aminoglycoside

The initial treatment of a neurosurgical patient with meningitis should include antibiotic coverage of staphylococci and gram-negative bacilli including *Klebsiella pneumoniae*, *Escherichia coli*, *Pseudomonas aeruginosa* and *Acinetobacter* species. *Streptococcus pneumoniae* is the most common cause of meningitis in the first few days following traumatic head injury. Therefore empiric antibiotic therapy for meningitis that develops in this setting should include coverage for *S. pneumoniae*. A third-generation cephalosporin is recommended for the treatment of gram-negative bacillary meningitis. Ceftazidime should be used because it is the only cephalosporin with sufficient activity against *P. aeruginosa* in the CNS. *Pseudomonas aeruginosa* meningitis should be treated with ceftazidime plus an aminoglycoside (gentamicin or tobramycin 240–360 mg/day in divided doses every 8 hours) for the first week of therapy.[1] The intraventricular administration of amino-glycosides is rarely indicated and should be reserved for cases of gram-negative meningitis where clinical improvement does not occur with intravenous antibiotic therapy.

Table 44.1 Antimicrobial therapy of bacterial meningitis in the neurosurgical patient

Etiology and organism	Antibiotic Total daily dose (dosing interval)
Cerebrospinal fluid shunt infection staphylococci	Oxacillin 9–12 g/day intravenously (every 4 h) *or* Vancomycin 2 g/day intravenously (every 6 h) *plus* Oral rifampin 1200 mg/day + / − Intrashunt or intraventricular vancomycin 20 mg once/day
Closed head injury *Streptococcus pneumoniae,* *Staphylococcus aureus,* *Haemophilus influenzae*	Ceftriaxone 2–4 g/day intravenously (every 12 h) *or* Cefotaxime 8 g/day intravenously (every 4 h) *plus* Vancomycin 2 g/day (every 6 h)
Gram-negative bacilli (except *Pseudomonas aeruginosa*) *Pseudomonas aeruginosa*	Ceftriaxone or cefotaxime Ceftazidime 6 g/day intravenously (every 8 h) *plus* Aminogylcoside for the first week of therapy
Streptococcus pneumoniae	Ceftriaxone *or* cefotaxime

Source: Tunkel AR, Scheld WM. Acute meningitis. In: Stein JH (ed.), *Internal medicine.* 4th edn. St Louis: Mosby, 1994; 1886–99.

Staphylococcus aureus and coagulase-negative staphylococci are the predominant organisms causing CSF shunt infections. Vancomycin is recommended for shunt infections due to staphylococci, unless the organism is clearly susceptible to methicillin. Therapy of CSF shunt infections due to methicillin-resistant staphylococci should include a combination of intravenous vancomycin and oral rifampin. Intrashunt or intraventricular vancomycin is added if the spinal fluid continues to yield viable organisms after 48 hours of intravenous therapy. Table 44.1 lists antimicrobial therapy in the neurosurgical patient by type of infection (CSF shunt infections), etiology (closed head injury), and the most likely infecting organisms (gram-negative bacilli, *S. pneumoniae*).

References

1. Fong IW, Tomkins KB. Review of *Pseudomonas aeruginosa* meningitis with special emphasis on treatment with ceftazidime. *Rev Infect Dis* 1985; **7**: 604–12.

45.   *Empiric therapy of bacterial meningitis in the immunocompromised patient is based on the type of immune abnormality*

Meningitis in neutropenic patients is usually due to the enteric gram-negative bacilli that reside in the gastrointestinal tract, *Pseudomonas aeruginosa*, *Escherichia coli*, *Klebsiella* and *Enterobacter* species. These patients are also at risk for meningitis due to hematogenous dissemination of *Staphylococcus aureus* and coagulase-negative staphylococci infections of hyperalimentation and other central intravenous lines. Empiric antimicrobial therapy of bacterial meningitis in neutropenic patients should include a combination of a third-generation cephalosporin (ceftazidime for *P. aeruginosa*) and vancomycin.

In individuals with a defect in cell-mediated immunity involving T-lymphocytes and macrophages of the type that occurs in patients with AIDS, organ transplant recipients, those with lymphomas and lymphocytic leukemias, and in patients receiving immunosuppressive doses of adrenocorticosteroids, *Listeria monocytogenes* is the most common causative organism of bacterial meningitis. Empiric therapy of meningitis in this group of patients should include ampicillin. The third-generation cephalosporins are inactive against *Listeria*.

Individuals with chronic lymphocytic leukemia, multiple myeloma, Hodgkin's disease, congenital or acquired hypogammaglobulinema and splenectomy have a decreased ability to mount an antibody response to a bacterial challenge, and are at risk for meningitis due to the encapsulated bacteria, *Streptococcus pneumoniae*, *Haemophilus influenzae* type b and *Neisseria meningitidis*. Empiric therapy of bacterial meningitis in these individuals should be with a third-generation cephalosporin, either ceftriaxone or cefotaxime. Due to the occurrence of penicillin-resistant pneumococcal meningitis, and the fact that bacterial meningitis in these patients can be rapidly fulminant, penicillin therapy is not recommended as empiric therapy for patients with this type of immune system abnormality. Table 45.1 lists empiric therapy of bacterial meningitis in immunocompromised patients based on the type of immune abnormality.

Table 45.1   Empiric therapy of bacterial meningitis in immunocompromised patients

Type of immune abnormality	Antibiotic Total daily dose (dosing interval)

Neutropenia (<1000/mm³) due to:
  Chemotherapy
  Radiotherapy
  Leukemia
  Aplastic anemia
	Ceftriaxone 2–4 g/day intravenously
	  (every 12 h)
	or
	Cefotaxime 8 g/day intravenously
	  (every 4 h)
	or
	Ceftazidime 6 g/day intravenously
	  (every 8 h)
	plus
	Vancomycin 2 g/day intravenously
	  (every 6 h)

T-lymphocyte and macrophage
defects due to:
  Acquired immune deficiency
  syndrome (AIDS)
  Organ transplantation
  Lymphomas
  Adrenocorticosteroid therapy
	Ampicillin 12 g/day intravenously
	  (every 4 h)

Immunoglobulin deficiency due to:
  Chronic lymphocytic leukemia
  Multiple myeloma
  Splenectomy
	Ceftriaxone *or* cefotaxime

Source: Pruitt AA. Central nervous system infections in cancer patients. *Neurol Clin* 1991; **9**, 867–88.

46.   *The American Academy of Pediatrics recommends consideration of dexamethasone therapy for bacterial meningitis in infants and children 2 months of age and older*

In 1988, Lebel et al.[1] published the results of two prospective double-blind placebo-controlled trials involving 200 infants and children (≥ 2 months old) to evaluate the efficacy of dexamethasone therapy in bacterial meningitis. The etiologic organism of bacterial meningitis was *Haemophilus influenzae* type b (Hib) in 154 cases. In each trial, 51 patients received dexamethasone (0.15 mg/kg body weight every 6 hours for 4 days) and 49 received placebo, in addition to antibiotic therapy. The patients in the first study group were treated with cefuroxime and the patients in the second study group were treated with ceftriaxone.

The administration of dexamethasone had a beneficial effect on the inflammatory profile of the CSF in the first 24 hours of therapy. The mean CSF glucose concentration in patients given dexamethasone increased 126% after 24 hours, compared with 26% in placebo recipients ($P<0.001$). Dexamethasone also had a beneficial effect on the protein concentration in the CSF. The mean decrease in the protein concentration after 24 hours of therapy was significantly greater in those who received dexamethasone than in the control group (64.0 versus 25.3 mg/dL).

The most striking result from this investigation, however, was the effect dexamethasone therapy had on sensorineural hearing loss. Dexamethasone significantly reduced the frequency of moderate, severe or profound bilateral sensorineural hearing loss. Thirteen of 84 patients (15.5%) in the placebo group had moderate or more severe bilateral hearing impairment as compared with 3 of 92 (3.3%) of the dexamethasone recipients ($P<0.01$). The beneficial effect of dexamethasone on hearing was documented for children with *H. influenzae* meningitis only; there were too few patients with pneumococcal or meningococcal meningitis to assess the efficacy of dexamethasone therapy in meningitis due to these organisms. In the dexamethasone-treated group, there were 79 cases of Hib meningitis, 8 cases of *Streptococcus pneumoniae* meningitis, 9 cases of meningococcal meningitis, 2 cases of group B streptococcus meningitis, and 4 cases in which the meningeal pathogen was not isolated. Two dexamethasone-treated infants had gastrointestinal (GI) bleeding. This complication occurred on the second and third days of dexamethasone therapy and required blood transfusion. It is not certain, however, whether or not the GI bleeding was the result of dexamethasone therapy. Dexamethasone therapy did not adversely affect the penetration of cefuroxime or ceftriaxone into the CSF, and did not affect the rate of sterilization of CSF cultures. All CSF cultures were sterile after 48 hours of therapy.[1]

Odio et al.[2] conducted a placebo-controlled, double-blind trial of dexamethasone therapy in 101 infants and children with bacterial meningitis in Costa Rica. Dexamethasone was given in the same dose as it was given in the studies by Lebel et al.[1] with the initial dose of dexamethasone being administered 15–20 minutes before the first dose of cefotaxime. In the dexamethasone-treated group of 52 infants and children, meningitis was due to Hib in 39 cases, *S. pneumoniae* in 4 cases, *Neisseria meningitidis* in 2 cases, and other meningeal pathogens in 7 cases. The results of this study demonstrated a significant reduction in meningeal inflammation in the patients treated with dexamethasone compared with the patients given placebo. By 12 hours of therapy, all indexes of inflammation in the CSF (CSF lactate, leukocytes, glucose and protein concentrations) had improved with dexamethasone therapy, whereas they had uniformly worsened in the patients given placebo. Neurologic sequelae occurred significantly more often in the patients who were given placebo.[2]

Girgis et al.[3] found a beneficial effect of dexamethasone on mortality from pneumococcal meningitis. In this clinical trial, 210 patients were treated with dexamethasone intramuscularly (8 mg to children younger than 12 years and 12 mg to adults every 12 hours for 3 days) in addition to ampicillin and chloramphenicol therapy. Two hundred and nineteen patients received antibiotics alone. One hundred and thirty-three patients in the dexamethasone-treated group and 140 patients in the group treated with antibiotics alone were comatose at the time of hospitalization. Dexamethasone was administered concomitantly with the first dose of antibiotic.

The case fatality rate was significantly lower in patients receiving dexamethasone; 20 of 210 patients treated with antibiotics and dexamethasone died, compared with 42 of 219 receiving antibiotics alone ($P<0.01$). This reduction was significantly different for patients with S. pneumoniae meningitis; 7 of 52 (13.5%) of the patients treated with antibiotics and dexamethasone died compared with 22 of 54 (40.7%) of the patients treated with antibiotics alone ($P<0.002$). The permanent neurologic sequelae seen on discharge and during the 6 month follow-up was reduced in patients treated with dexamethasone, but significant benefit occurred only in patients with S. pneumoniae meningitis. None of the 45 surviving patients in the dexamethasone-treated group developed hearing loss, whereas 4 of 32 in the group treated with antibiotics alone became deaf ($P<0.05$). The investigators were unable to evaluate hearing loss in the children with H. influenzae meningitis because they were too young for conventional audiometric evaluation and brainstem evoked response audiometry (BAER) was not available.[3]

The results of these clinical trials prompted the American Academy of Pediatrics to take a stance on the use of dexamethasone therapy in bacterial meningitis in infants and children in 1990. The Committee recommended the consideration of dexamethasone for bacterial meningitis in infants and children 2 months of age and older. The recommended dosage is 0.6 mg/kg/day in four divided doses (0.15 mg/kg/dose) given intravenously for the first 4 days of antibiotic treatment. In 1990 the Committee recommended that the first dose of dexamethasone be administered at the time of the first dose of antibacterial therapy but the present recommendation is to administer the first dose of dexamethasone 20 minutes prior to the first dose of antibacterial therapy.[4] Although the Committee recognized that the results of clinical trials had demonstrated a beneficial effect of dexamethasone therapy in reducing the incidence of deafness in H. influenzae meningitis, the Committee also stated in its report that the utility of dexamethasone therapy in the treatment of pneumococcal or meningococcal meningitis was not yet known.

In December 1991, Kennedy et al.[5] published the results of a review of the medical records of 97 infants and children with pneumococcal meningitis who were treated from 1984 to 1990. Forty-one patients received corticosteroid therapy, 39 of whom were given dexamethasone 0.15 mg/kg/dose every 6 hours for 4 days. Among the survivors, there were significantly fewer patients with an overall adverse neurologic outcome, including hearing impairment, in the group that received steroid therapy compared with the group that did not (4 of 35 versus 14 of 43). Twenty-seven of the 97 infants and children had evidence of fulminant meningeal infection. These patients were sicker than those without evidence of fulminant meningeal infection, as defined by laboratory studies, altered level of consciousness, the presence of septic shock, cerebrovascular instability and GI bleeding. They accounted for two-thirds of the deaths and had a significantly increased incidence of seizures and permanent bilateral moderate or greater hearing loss. Of the survivors of overwhelming meningeal infection, 1 of 8 steroid-treated patients compared with 7 of 13 non-steroid-treated patients had moderate or greater bilateral hearing loss. The 1 steroid-treated patient had severe neurologic damage and BAER evidence of bilateral hearing loss before dexamethasone therapy was administered 31 hours after the first parenteral dose of antibiotics.[5]

Schaad et al.[6] published the results of a prospective, placebo-controlled, double-blind trial of dexamethasone in 115 children with acute bacterial meningitis in Switzerland. Dexamethasone therapy (0.4 mg/kg) was started 10 minutes before the first dose of ceftriaxone and given every 12 hours for 2 days. After 24 hours of treatment, the increase in CSF glucose concentration was significantly greater in the dexamethasone group than in the placebo group. At follow-up examination 3, 9 and 15 months after hospital discharge, 3 of 60 (5%) dexamethasone recipients had one or more neurologic or audiologic sequelae compared with 9 of 55 (16%) placebo recipients ($P=0.066$). *Haemophilus influenzae* was the infecting organism in 30 of 55 patients (55%) in the placebo group, and in 37 of 60 (62%) of the patients in the dexamethasone-treated group. *Neisseria meningitidis* was the infecting organism in 12 of 55 patients (22%) in the placebo group, and 16 of 60 patients (27%) in the dexamethasone-treated group.[6]

A prospective double-blind placebo-controlled trial to evaluate the efficacy of dexamethasone therapy in adults with bacterial meningitis has not been published to date, but the pathophysiology of the neurologic complications of bacterial meningitis as described in chapter 2 is the same in children and adults. In the words of Sir William Osler: "In seeking absolute truth we aim at the unattainable, and must be content with finding broken portions".[7] In experimental models of meningitis, dexamethasone has been shown to decrease cerebral edema and intracranial pressure, to decrease the leakage of serum proteins into the CSF and to minimize the alteration in blood–brain barrier permeability. In experimental models of meningitis in rabbits, dexamethasone has been demonstrated to decrease the meningeal inflammatory response that is induced by the intracisternal injection of Hib endotoxin.[8] Syrogiannopoulos et al.[9] evaluated dexamethasone therapy in an experimental model of Hib meningitis. Dexamethasone in combination with ceftriaxone reduced the brain water content in infected animals to a greater degree than did ceftriaxone alone. Dexamethasone alone or in combination with ceftriaxone decreased intracranial pressure to a greater degree than ceftriaxone alone.

The results of clinical and experimental studies in addition to our knowledge of the pathophysiology of bacterial meningitis leads to the recommendation that the use of dexamethasone therapy be considered for adults with bacterial meningitis. The recommended dose of dexamethasone is 0.6 mg/kg/day in four divided doses (0.15 mg/kg/dose) given intravenously for the first 4 days of antimicrobial therapy. Dexamethasone should be administered 20 minutes prior to the first dose of antibiotic. The reason for giving dexamethasone prior to the first dose of antibiotic is based on the

PATHOPHYSIOLOGY OF BACTERIAL MENINGITIS

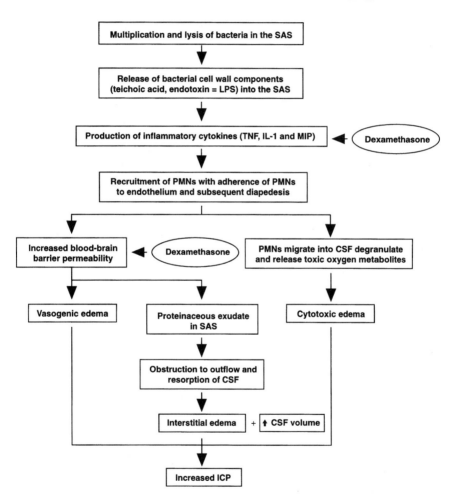

SAS = Subarachnoid Space, LPS = Lipopolysaccharide, TNF = Tumor Necrosis Factor ∝,
IL-1 = Interleukin-1, MIP = Macrophage Inflammatory Protein, ICP = Intracranial Pressure

Fig. 46.1   Dexamethasone decreases cerebral edema and intracranial pressure by inhibiting the production of inflammatory cytokines and by minimizing the alteration in blood–brain barrier permeability.

results of experimental studies. In the experimental model of meningitis used by Mustafa[8] (described above), dexamethasone was given intravenously 1 hour before, at the same time as, and 30 minutes after the intracisternal injection of 20 ng Hib lipooligosaccharide (LOS; endotoxin). Dexamethasone administered 1 hour before or simultaneously with LOS inoculation was associated with significantly lower CSF tumor necrosis factor (TNF), protein and lactate concentrations, and higher CSF glucose concentrations, compared with those of animals that received dexamethasone 30 minutes after LOS inoculation and of animals given LOS alone. There was also a significantly lower white blood cell (WBC) count in the CSF of rabbits treated with dexamethasone at the time of induction of meningitis compared with control rabbits. When dexamethasone was administered 30 minutes after intracisternal LOS administration, there was no significant effect on CSF WBC counts or on glucose, protein and lactate concentrations when compared with values obtained in control animals. This is explained by the mechanism by which dexamethasone has an inhibitory effect on TNF production. In studies *in vitro*, dexamethasone inhibits the production of TNF if administered to macrophages before they are activated by endotoxin, both by diminishing the quantity of TNF mRNA that is produced in response to endotoxin and by preventing its translation. Dexamethasone is unable to regulate TNF production once induction has occurred.[8] As has been discussed in chapter 2, the initiation of antibiotic therapy results in the lysis of bacterial organisms with the release of free endotoxin into the CSF. The timing of the administration of dexamethasone to coincide with the release of endotoxin allows dexamethasone to inhibit TNF production and limit the inflammatory cascade that follows (Fig. 46.1).

References

1. Lebel MH, Freij BT, Syrogiannopoulos GA et al. Dexamethasone therapy for bacterial meningitis: results of two double-blind, placebo-controlled trials. *N Engl J Med* 1988; **319:** 964–71.
2. Odio CM, Faingezicht I, Paris M, Nassar M. The beneficial effects of early dexamethasone administration in infants and children with bacterial meningitis. *N Engl J Med* 1991; **324:** 1525–31.
3. Girgis NI, Farid Z, Mikhail IA et al. Dexamethasone treatment for bacterial meningitis in children and adults. *Pediatr Infect Dis J* 1989; **8:** 848–51.
4. Committee on Infectious Diseases. Dexamethasone therapy for bacterial meningitis in infants and children. *Pediatrics* 1990; **86:** 130–3.
5. Kennedy WA, Hoyt MJ, McCracken GH. The role of corticosteroid therapy in children with pneumococcal meningitis. *Am J Dis Child* 1991; **145:** 1374–8.
6. Schaad UB, Lips U, Gnehm HE et al. Dexamethasone therapy for bacterial meningitis in children. *Lancet* 1993; **342:** 457–61.
7. Osler W. Aequanimitas. Valedictory Address, University of Pennsylvania, May 1, 1889. In: Reynolds R, Stone J (eds), *On Doctoring.* New York: Simon and Schuster, 1991; 32–8.

8. Mustafa MM, Ramilo O, Olsen KD, et al. Tumor necrosis factor in mediating experimental *Haemophilus influenzae* type b meningitis. *J Clin Invest* 1989; **84:** 1253–9.
9. Syrogiannopoulos GA, Olsen KD, Reisch JS, McCracken GH. Dexamethasone in the treatment of experimental *Haemophilus influenzae* type b meningitis. *J Infect Dis* 1987; **155:** 213–39.

47. *The concomitant use of an H_2-antagonist with dexamethasone is recommended to avoid the most serious complication of dexamethasone therapy*

The most serious adverse effect of dexamethasone therapy is gastrointestinal (GI) bleeding. In the clinical trials in Dallas, 2 of the 102 dexamethasone-treated patients had GI bleeding. In both cases, the bleeding occurred 2–3 days after admission, the coagulation studies were normal, and transfusions of blood products were required. One patient had *Haemophilus influenzae* meningitis and had hypotension, apnea and acidosis on admission to the hospital. The second patient had pneumococcal meningitis and had been followed for gastroenteritis in the week before admission, during which time he had an unexplained decline of 40 g/L in hemoglobin concentration. Two additional patients who received dexamethasone and ceftriaxone had heme-positive stools without overt bleeding.[1]

In another clinical trial of dexamethasone therapy in 100 infants and children with bacterial meningitis, heme-positive stools were detected in 12 of 51 (24%) dexamethasone-treated patients and in 21 of 48 (44%) patients treated with antibiotics alone. This is an interesting finding suggesting perhaps that the stress of the central nervous system disease is more likely to be responsible for the heme-positive stools than the dexamethasone therapy.

In the review by Kennedy et al.[2] of the records of 97 infants and children with pneumococcal meningitis, 4 patients in each of the steroid- and non-steroid-treated groups had clinically evident GI bleeding, and 3 patients in each group required a blood transfusion. Two patients in each group had evidence of blood loss before diagnosis and treatment. Two patients with GI bleeding died; both were from the non-steroid-treated group. All patients with clinically apparent GI bleeding had an altered sensorium, either obtundation or coma on admission, and all but one had evidence of sepsis or septic shock.

In a clinical trial of dexamethasone therapy in 115 children with acute bacterial meningitis, there were no cases of overt GI bleeding, but occult-blood tests on stool were positive in 11 of 39 (28%) dexamethasone-treated and 4 of 31 (13%) placebo-treated patients on day 3, and in 10 of 49 (20%) dexamethasone-treated patients and 5 of 43 (12%) placebo-treated patients at the end of treatment.[3] The concomitant use of an intravenous H_2-antagonist is recommended with dexamethasone therapy.

In the clinical trials in Dallas, dexamethasone did not affect the rate of sterilization of CSF cultures. All CSF cultures were sterile after 48 hours of therapy. Secondary fever, defined as a rectal temperature of at least 38.0°C after at least 24 hours of maximal daily temperatures of 37.9°C, occurred more frequently in the dexamethasone-treated patients. Secondary fever occurred in 63 of 102 (62%) dexamethasone-treated patients compared to 34 of 98 (35%) placebo-treated patients. The etiology of the secondary fever was not identified.[1] A secondary fever that develops in the course of acute bacterial meningitis may be due to a nosocomial viral illness, an infection at an intravenous access site, a drug reaction, a complication of the meningitis, or a failure of therapy.[4] Although secondary fever occurred more often in the dexamethasone-treated patients in the clinical trials in Dallas, the fever lasted less than 24 hours and was not associated with complications of meningitis. In another clinical trial of dexamethasone therapy in 101 infants and children with bacterial meningitis, secondary fever occurred with similar frequency in the dexamethasone- and placebo-treated groups. Prolonged fever (7 days or longer) occurred more frequently in the placebo group than in the dexamethasone group ($P<0.003$).[5]

In the clinical trials in Dallas, there was only one death and that was in the placebo-treated group, the result of late complications of H. influenzae meningitis.[1] In a clinical trial involving 101 infants and children with bacterial meningitis, there were two deaths, one in the dexamethasone-treated group and one in the placebo group. Subdural empyema associated with H. influenzae meningitis developed in one placebo recipient. Seizures developed after 48 hours of treatment in 2 of 51 (4%) patients given dexamethasone and in 7 of 48 (15%) given placebo.[5] In the review by Kennedy et al.[2] of the records of 97 infants and children with pneumococcal meningitis, there were four deaths in the steroid-treated group and five deaths in the non-steroid-treated group.

Perhaps the greatest concern among practitioners is the administration of dexamethasone to a patient who has a non-bacterial cause of meningitis. A short course of dexamethasone therapy should not adversely affect the outcome in patients with viral meningitis. Waagner et al.[6] found no adverse effects of dexamethasone therapy in patients with subsequently documented viral meningitis. This diagnosis is usually established within 24 hours based on the results of CSF examination and dexamethasone therapy can be discontinued at that time. The main argument against using dexamethasone in bacterial meningitis is that dexamethasone will decrease meningeal inflammation, and a moderate degree of meningeal inflammation is required for the CSF penetration of many antimicrobial agents. In clinical practice, however, dexamethasone has not affected the early rate of sterilization of CSF cultures.[1] Several days into treatment, however, when meningeal inflammation has been reduced substantially by dexamethasone, the penetration of antibiotics into CSF may be reduced. Dexamethasone therapy should, therefore, be discontinued after 4 days.

In cases of tuberculous meningitis, dexamethasone therapy is recommended when one of the following complications has developed:

1. altered consciousness;
2. papilledema;
3. focal neurologic deficit, and/or
4. CSF opening pressure >300 mmH$_2$O.[7]

The rationale for the use of dexamethasone in the setting of these complications is that the pathophysiology of altered consciousness and raised intracranial pressure is the same in acute tuberculous meningitis as in acute bacterial meningitis. In a large clinical trial, involving 280 patients with a clinical presentation of tuberculous meningitis, there was a significant reduction in mortality and neurologic complications, and a significantly more rapid normalization of the CSF white blood cell count, and protein and glucose concentrations, in the patients treated with dexamethasone plus antituberculous chemotherapy than in the patients treated with antituberculous chemotherapy alone.[8] The concomitant use of dexamethasone therapy is not presently recommended in patients with fungal meningitis, but clinical trials are underway.

References

1. Lebel MH, Freij BJ, Syrogiannopoulos GA, Chrane DF, et al. Dexamethasone therapy for bacterial meningitis: results of two double-blind, placebo-controlled trials. *N Engl J Med* 1988; **319**: 964–71.
2. Kennedy WA, Hoyt MJ, McCracken GH. The role of corticosteroid therapy in children with pneumococcal meningitis. *Am J Dis Child* 1991; **145**: 1374–8.
3. Schaad UB, Lips U, Gnehm HE, Blumberg A, et al. Dexamethasone therapy for bacterial meningitis in children. *Lancet* 1993; **342**: 457–61.
4. Feder HM. To the editor. *N Engl J Med* 1989; **320**: 465.
5. Odio CM, Faingezicht I, Paris M, Nassar M. The beneficial effects of early dexamethasone administration in infants and children with bacterial meningitis. *N Engl J Med* 1991; **324**: 1525–31.
6. Waagner DC, Kennedy WA, Hoyt MJ, McCracken GH Jr. Lack of adverse effects of dexamethasone therapy in aseptic meningitis. *Pediatr Infect Dis J* 1990; **10**: 922–3.
7. Molavi A, LeFrock JL. Tuberculous meningitis. *Med Clin North Amer* 1985; **69**: 315–31.
8. Girgis NI, Farid Z, Kilpatrick ME, Sultan Y, Mikhail IA. Dexamethasone adjunctive treatment for tuberculous meningitis. *Pediatr Infect Dis J* 1991; **10**: 179–83.

48.   *As leukocytes do more harm than good in the subarachnoid space, leukocyte monoclonal antibody therapy may prove valuable as adjunctive therapy for bacterial meningitis*

The use of antibodies for adjunctive therapy of bacterial meningitis is not an entirely new and revolutionary therapeutic approach to this infection. Early in this century, when the diagnosis of acute pyogenic meningitis was made, intrathecal antimeningococcus horse serum was administered immediately. With the availability of the sulfonamide compounds, the recognition that each microorganism has an antigenically distinct polysaccharide capsule, and the observation that antibodies formed by the host in response to the infection play a part in the recovery process, the treatment of choice became a combination of sulfadiazine and a type-specific rabbit antibody against the capsular polysaccharide of the infecting organism. The antisera was initially administered intravenously. The dosage of the antibody was determined by the degree of CSF hypoglycorrhachia based on the observation that the magnitude of hypoglycorrhachia correlated with the severity of the infection. If the patient failed to show satisfactory improvement after 48 hours of parenteral therapy, the intrathecal administration of antibody was recommended.[1]

Before entering the subarachnoid space, leukocytes must first adhere to cerebral capillary endothelial cells through a group of adhesion-promoting receptors and ligands located on leukocyte cell membranes and endothelial cells.[2] The adherence of leukocytes to endothelial cells is greatly increased by exposure to the inflammatory cytokines, interleukin-1 and tumor necrosis factor (TNF).[3] The endothelial leukocyte-adhesion molecule-1 (ELAM-1) is inducible on endothelial cells after stimulation with interleukin-1 and TNF.[4] Once in the subarachnoid space, leukocytes are more harmful than beneficial and do little to eradicate the infection in the subarachnoid space. The major defense function of leukocytes, the phagocytosis of microorganisms, is inefficient in a fluid medium.[5] Leukocytes are, however, harmful to the host. Large numbers of leukocytes in the subarachnoid space contribute to the purulent exudate and obstruct the flow of CSF. The adherence of leukocytes to cerebral capillary endothelial cells increases the permeability of blood vessels, allowing the leakage of plasma proteins through open intercellular junctions leading to vasogenic brain edema. The leukocytes that successfully migrate into the CSF can subsequently be stimulated by the inflammatory cytokines, TNF and interleukin-1, to degranulate and release toxic oxygen metabolites producing cytotoxic cerebral edema. Cytotoxic cerebral edema contributes to the encephalopathy of bacterial meningitis.[6]

The predominant mechanism of leukocyte migration across the blood–brain barrier involves the CD11/CD18 receptors on leukocytes. In an experimental model of bacterial meningitis, rabbits were injected intracisternally with pneumococci. Treatment was then initiated with ampicillin and, in one group, antibody therapy directed against the CD11/CD18 receptors on leukocytes was also given. Antibody-treated animals had significantly less leukocytosis and protein accumulation in the CSF than control animals. Bacterial killing by ampicillin was equivalent in the antibody-treated and control animals. Three of 4 control animals died in contrast to none of the 11 antibody-treated animals. The investigators concluded that:

1. bacteria do not have an advantage for growth in the absence of functional neutrophils in the CSF;
2. therapy with leukocyte monoclonal antibodies and the resultant decrease in inflammation improved survival, provided bacterial killing was achieved by adequate antibiotic therapy.[5]

Figure 48.1 demonstrates where leukocyte monoclonal antibody therapy would alter the pathophysiology of bacterial meningitis.

PATHOPHYSIOLOGY OF BACTERIAL MENINGITIS

SAS = Subarachnoid Space, LPS = Lipopolysaccharide, TNF = Tumor Necrosis Factor ∝,
IL-1 = Interleukin-1, MIP = Macrophage Inflammatory Protein, ICP = Intracranial Pressure

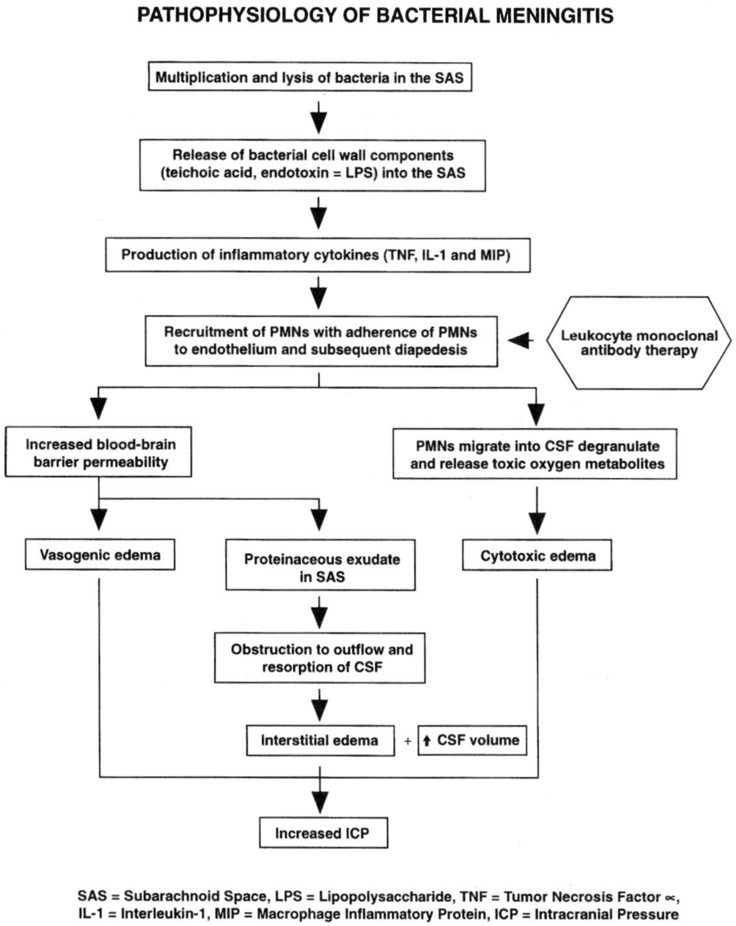

Fig. 48.1   Leukocyte monoclonal antibody therapy limits the inflammatory cascade at the step marked.

A combination of dexamethasone and anti-CD18 monoclonal antibodies was used to determine whether this would be more effective than either agent used alone in reducing meningeal inflammation in experimental *Haemophilus influenzae* type b (Hib) meningitis.[2] Dexamethasone was used because of its ability to inhibit the production of interleukin-1 and TNF. Experimental evidence suggests that TNF and interleukin have a role in the activation of the CD11 and CD18 receptor complexes, suggesting that the interaction of cytokine, endothelium and leukocyte is responsible for the disruption of the blood–brain barrier, and the passage of serum proteins into the subarachnoid space.[7] In experimental Hib meningitis, the combination of dexamethasone and anti-CD11/CD18 antibodies was more effective than either agent used alone in reducing the influx of neutrophils and protein into the CSF.[2] The advantage of the leukocyte monoclonal antibody therapy over anti-cytokine or antibacterial antibody therapy is that the leukocyte monoclonal antibody therapy can be given intravenously to keep circulating leukocytes out of the CSF. In contrast, the other antibodies must be given intrathecally because they do not cross an uninflamed or inflamed blood–brain barrier well.[5]

References

1. Alexander HE. Treatment of *Haemophilus influenzae* infection and of meningococcic and pneumococcic meningitis. *Am J Dis Child* 1943; **66:** 172–87.
2. Saez-Llorens X, Jafari HS, Severien C, et al. Enhanced attenuation of meningeal inflammation and brain edema by concomitant administration of anti-CD18 monoclonal antibodies and dexamethasone in experimental *Haemophilus* meningitis. *J Clin Invest* 1991; **88:** 2003–11.
3. Moser R, Schleiffenbaum B, Groscurth P, Fehr J. Interleukin 1 and tumor necrosis factor stimulate human vascular endothelial cells to promote transendothelial neutrophil passage. *J Clin Invest* 1989; **83:** 444–55.
4. Quagliarello V, Scheld WM. Bacterial meningitis: pathogenesis, pathophysiology, and progress. *N Engl J Med* 1992; **327:** 864–72.
5. Tuomanen E, Baruch A. New antibodies as adjunctive therapies for gram-positive bacterial meningitis. *Pediatr Infect Dis J* 1989; **8:** 923–8.
6. Fishman RA, Sligar K, Hake RB. Effects of leukocytes on brain metabolism in granulocytic brain edema. *Ann Neurol* 1977; **2:** 89–94.
7. Springer TA. Adhesion receptors of the immune system. *Nature* 1990; **364:** 425–33.

49.   *If IgG monoclonal antibodies are to be valuable for adjunctive therapy of bacterial meningitis, the direct intracisternal inoculation of the antibodies is necessary*

As was discussed in maxim 48, in the early part of this century, the treatment of choice for bacterial meningitis was a combination of sulfadiazine and a type-specific rabbit antibody against the capsular polysaccharide of the infecting organism. The best clinical response was achieved when the antisera was administered intrathecally.[1] There is renewed interest in using monoclonal antibody therapy in bacterial meningitis. However, formulations of mouse or rabbit monoclonal antibodies that possess therapeutic activity against the bacteria most frequently causing bacteremia in neonates and adults have had serious shortcomings when administered to humans. Human antibodies will react with foreign mouse or rabbit antibodies and accelerate mouse or rabbit antibody clearance. There is also an increased likelihood of developing a serum sickness-like syndrome.[2,3] For these reasons, human monoclonal antibodies to specific bacterial pathogens would be superior therapeutic agents. Human monoclonal antibodies have been produced that demonstrate specific reactivity to the K1 capsule of *Escherichia coli* and the group B polysaccharide of *Neisseria meningitidis*. Although these antibodies enhanced opsonophagocytic activity *in vitro*, the antibody caused bacterial removal only in the presence of human complement and neutrophils. As the CSF is an area of complement deficiency, human monoclonal antibody therapy would have to be administered together with complement. Monoclonal antibodies to meningococcal lipopolysaccharides were highly protective against bacterial challenge in an infant rat model of meningococcal infection.[4]

There are at least two limitations to using human monoclonal antibody therapy in the treatment of bacterial meningitis. Using a rabbit model of meningitis, Gigliotti et al.[5] examined the ability of a human monoclonal antibody to enter the CSF. By measuring the anti-binding capacity of the human monoclonal antibody present in simultaneous serum and CSF samples, the investigators were able to determine the proportion of functional IgG in serum that is able to penetrate into the CSF. The results of this investigation suggested that, even during active inflammation, the blood–brain barrier is an effective barrier to antibody penetration into the CSF. To achieve sufficient antibody concentrations within the CSF, it would be necessary to produce serum concentrations of antibodies of at least 20–100-fold higher than the expected protective concentration in serum.[5] To achieve protective concentrations of antibody in the CSF, intrathecal injection would be required. The second limitation to using monoclonal antibody therapy to treat bacterial meningitis is the deficiency of complement in the CSF. Complement is likely to be required for the optimal function of intrathecally administered antibody, and may have to be administered with the antibody. It is not yet known whether there is sufficient complement in the CSF for the optimal function of antibody therapy.[5]

Immunoglobulin G (IgG) monoclonal antibodies to the inflammatory cytokines should theoretically be valuable as adjunctive therapy for bacterial meningitis. The inflammatory cytokines, macrophage inflammatory protein 1 (MIP-1) and macrophage inflammatory protein 2 (MIP-2) induce an influx of polymorphonuclear leukocytes into the CSF. Antibodies to either MIP-1 or MIP-2 cause a significant delay in the leukocytosis induced by pneumococci, IL-1 or tumor necrosis factor (TNF), indicating that these inflammatory cytokines take part in recruiting leukocytes in meningitis.[6] The practical disadvantage of IgG monoclonal antibody to human recombinant interleukin-1 or TNF is that, by the time the diagnosis of bacterial meningitis is made, these inflammatory cytokines are present in the subarachnoid space. In addition, the release of bacterial cell wall components by bacteriolytic antibiotics stimulates the production of these inflammatory cytokines. Monoclonal antibody therapy directed against the inflammatory cytokines that is given either before or concomitantly with antibiotic therapy would potentially be beneficial. Any therapeutic modality, however, that requires intrathecal administration is problematic in bacterial meningitis because of the frequent occurrence of raised intracranial pressure and the risks of administering intrathecal therapy in this setting.

References

1. Alexander HE. Treatment of *Haemophilus influenzae* infections and of meningococcic and pneumococcic meningitis. *Am J Dis Child* 1943; **66:** 172–87.
2. Levy R, Miller RA. Tumor therapy with monoclonal antibodies. *Fed Proc* 1983; **42:** 2650–6.
3. Raff HV, Devereux D, Shuford W, Abbott-Brown D, Maloney G. Human monoclonal antibody with protective activity for *Echerichia coli* K1 and *Neisseria meningitidis* group B infections. *J Infect Dis* 1988; **157:** 118–26.
4. Saukkonen K, Leinonen M, Kayhty H, Abdillahi H, Poolman JT. Monoclonal antibodies to the rough lipopolysaccharide of *Neisseria meningitidis* protect infant rats from meningococcal infection. *J Infect Dis* 1988; **158:** 209–11.
5. Gigliotti F, Lee D, Insel RA, Scheld WM. IgG penetration into the cerebrospinal fluid in a rabbit model of meningitis. *J Infect Dis* 1987; **156:** 394–8.
6. Tuomanen E, Baruch A. New antibodies as adjunctive therapies for gram-positive bacterial meningitis. *Pediatr Infect Dis J* 1989; **8:** 923–8.

50.   *Pentoxifylline decreases the adherence of neutrophils, which have been activated by inflammatory cytokines, to cerebral capillary endothelial cells*

Pentoxifylline (Trental) is a phosphodiesterase inhibitor that decreases platelet adhesion and aggregation, increases red cell deformability, reduces blood viscosity, and has been used for several years in the treatment of intermittent claudication from occlusive peripheral vascular disease. It has also been used in clinical trials for stroke. Pentoxifylline and its metabolites decrease the adherence of neutrophils that have been activated by interleukin-1 (IL-1) and tumor necrosis factor (TNF) to capillary endothelial cells, and decrease superoxide production and the rate of granule enzyme release on stimulation.[1] The inhibitory effect that pentoxifylline has on neutrophils *in vitro* is most marked when the neutrophils have been pre-exposed to the inflammatory cytokines, TNF and IL-1.[2] Pentoxifylline significantly reduced the peak concentrations of leukocytes and lactate in CSF when administered 1 hour after intracisternal inoculation of endotoxin, by attenuating cytokine-induced leukocyte-endothelium interactions. Pentoxifylline treatment (initially an intravenous injection of 20 ng/kg followed by 6 mg/kg/h) started 20 minutes before intracisternal injection of 20 ng of *Haemophilus influenzae* type b (Hib) lipooligosaccharide (endotoxin) significantly reduced concentrations of leukocytes, protein and lactate in CSF during the 9 hour infusion compared with values in intravenous-saline-treated rabbits. When pentoxifylline was given 1 hour after Hib endotoxin, the mean peak lactate and leukocyte concentrations in CSF were significantly lower than those in control animals.[2] The latter observation suggests that pentoxifylline is beneficial even when given well into the course of the inflammatory cascade.

In a second group of experiments, rabbits were inoculated intracisternally with 2×10^4 colony-forming units of live Hib organisms. At 6 hours, rabbits were treated intravenously with one of four different regimens: saline, saline plus dexamethasone, pentoxifylline or dexamethasone plus pentoxifylline. Thirty minutes later all rabbits received ceftriaxone (100 mg/kg) and were followed for a further 6 hours. Pentoxifylline significantly decreased CSF lactate and protein concentrations, and decreased polymorphonuclear leukocyte counts compared with results in control animals. Dexamethasone, however, was superior to pentoxifylline in decreasing the meningeal inflammatory response, and no synergism was observed when the drugs were combined in these experiments.[3]

Pentoxifylline attenuated meningeal inflammatory changes induced by intracisternal inoculation of 10 ng of rabbit recombinant interleukin-1 beta compared with results in either dexamethasone- or saline-treated animals. In this latter experiment, pentoxifylline was superior to dexamethasone in reducing meningeal inflammation, suggesting that pentoxifylline could be effective in later stages of the inflammatory cascade even when cytokines are already produced and present in the CSF.[3]

References

1. Sullivan GW, Carper HT, Novick WJ, Mandell GL. Inhibition of the inflammatory action of interleukin-1 and tumor necrosis factor (alpha) on neutrophil function by pentoxifylline. *Infect Immun* 1988; **56:** 1722–9.
2. Saez-Llorens X, Ramilo O, Mustafa MM, Mertsola J, et al. Pentoxifylline modulates meningeal inflammation in experimental bacterial meningitis. *Antimicrob Agents Chemo* 1990; **34:** 837–43.
3. Saez-Llorens X, Ramilo O, Mustafa MM, Mertsola J. Modulation of meningeal inflammation by treatment with pentoxifylline. *Pediatr Infect Dis J* 1989; **8:** 922–3.

51.   Nonsteroidal anti-inflammatory agents reduce prostaglandin E_2 concentrations in CSF, reduce the influx of leukocytes and protein into CSF, reduce brain edema, but do not reduce intracranial pressure

Tumor necrosis factor and interleukin-1 stimulate the production of metabolites of arachidonic acid (AA), most notably prostaglandin E_2 (PGE$_2$) and prostacyclin (PGI$_2$). Prostaglandin E_2, a vasodilator, in combination with other inflammatory mediators, is known to increase vascular permeability and promote the leakage of plasma proteins into the subarachnoid space.[1] The anti-inflammatory properties of the nonsteroidal anti-inflammatory agents reside in their ability to inhibit the cyclooxygenase enzyme, thus preventing the conversion of arachidonic acid to biologically active prostaglandins (PGE$_2$ and PGI$_2$).[2]

In an experimental model of pneumococcal meningitis, the effect of inhibitors of the arachidonic acid metabolic pathways on the degree of inflammation in the subarachnoid space (leukocyte counts and protein concentration) was investigated. The most effective inhibitors of the inflammatory response were methylprednisolone and the cyclooxygenase inhibitor, oxindanac, which decreased the number of leukocytes by more than 90%. The cyclooxygenase inhibitors, diclofenac sodium and indomethacin, also reduced inflammation, but not as effectively as methylprednisolone and oxindanac. The effects of oxindanac and indomethacin were dose-dependent. As the dose of drug was decreased, the mean number of leukocytes present in CSF increased toward control values. Oxindanac was far superior to indomethacin in reducing meningeal inflammation. When repeated intracisternal doses of pneumococcal cell walls were administered to rabbits that were pretreated orally with oxindanac 1 hour before cell wall challenge, the influx of polymorphonuclear leukocytes was significantly less than in control animals. Oxindanac also decreased the incidence of severe meningeal signs such as paralysis and death in the experimental animals. To determine if the anti-inflammatory effects of cyclooxygenase inhibitors would modulate the inflammation associated with bacterial lysis *in vivo*, oxindanac and ampicillin were used to treat animals with established pneumococcal meningitis. The number of leukocytes appearing in CSF after a dose of ampicillin was significantly lower in the animals that also received oxindanac. Oxindanac did not alter the concentration of ampicillin in the CSF. Effective bacterial killing occurred in oxindanac-treated animals despite the lower density of CSF leukocytes.[3]

In an experimental model of pneumococcal meningitis in rabbits, a massive influx of serum albumin into the CSF, as well as other proteins of high and low molecular weight, was observed during the acute phase of meningitis. The administration of ampicillin with either dexamethasone or oxindanac was partially effective in preventing the alterations in CSF protein concentration during the acute phase of the infection. A rapid resolution of the abnormal pattern of CSF protein, including albumin, was also seen in animals treated with either dexamethasone or oxindanac but not in untreated animals or those given monotherapy with ampicillin.[4]

In experimental models of pneumococcal meningitis, indomethacin decreases PGE_2 concentrations in CSF, and decreases cytotoxic brain edema, but it does not significantly decrease intracranial pressure.[4,5]

One of the limitations of the use of nonsteroidal anti-inflammatory agents in the therapy of bacterial meningitis is that these agents must be given orally. A parenteral formulation is not available at the present time. As has been described in Chapter 3, a great many patients will be either stuporous or comatose at the time of presentation or shortly thereafter. Medications that require oral administration are undesirable when stupor or coma are present. In addition, the biological activities of PGE_2 are beneficial as well as detrimental to the individual. Prostaglandin E_2 appears to inhibit chemotaxis of polymorphonuclear leukocytes in response to immune complexes and inhibits the degranulation of leukocytes.[6,7] These properties would be beneficial to the patient. There is also experimental evidence to suggest that a reduction in CSF PGE_2 concentrations by indomethacin may allow for an influx of leukocytes into CSF.[8] The role of nonsteroidal anti-inflammatory agents in the treatment of acute bacterial meningitis has not been investigated in clinical trials. These agents are, however, efficacious in the reduction of fever. Oxindanac is superior to indomethacin in reducing meningeal inflammation.[3] The benefit or lack of benefit of a nonsteroidal anti-inflammatory agent on the outcome of bacterial meningitis may depend on the specific agent chosen for investigation. As has been demonstrated in experimental models of meningitis, all nonsteroidal anti-inflammatory agents are not equally efficacious in reducing meningeal inflammation. As this class of agents reduces brain edema but does not reduce intracranial pressure, their role as adjunctive agents in the therapy of bacterial meningitis has obvious limitations.

References

1. Kadurugamuwa JL, Hengstler B, Zak O. Effects of anti-inflammatory drugs on arachidonic acid metabolites and cerebrospinal fluid proteins during infectious pneumococcal meningitis in rabbits. *Pediatr Infect Dis J* 1987; **6**: 1153–4.
2. Saez-Llorens X, Ramilo O, Mustafa MM, Mertsola J, McCracken GH. Molecular pathophysiology of bacterial meningitis: current concepts and therapeutic implications. *J Pediatr* 1990; **116**: 671–84.
3. Tuomanen E, Hengstler B, Rich R, Bray MA, Zak O, Tomasz A. Nonsteroidal anti-inflammatory agents in the therapy for experimental pneumococcal meningitis. *J Infect Dis* 1987; **155**: 985–90.
4. Kadurugamuwa JL, Hengstler B, Zak O. Cerebrospinal fluid protein profile in experimental pneumococcal meningitis and its alteration by ampicillin and anti-inflammatory agents. *J Infect Dis* 1989; **159**: 26–33.

5. Tureen JH, Tauber MG, Sande MA. Effect of indomethacin on the pathophysiology of experimental meningitis in rabbits. *J Infect Dis* 1991; **163:** 647–9.
6. Fantone JC, Marasco WA, Elgas LJ, Ward PA. Anti-inflammatory effects of prostaglandin E_1: *in vivo* modulation of the formyl peptide chemotactic receptor on the rat neutrophil. *J Immunol* 1983; **130:** 1495–7.
7. Kaplan HB, Edelson HS, Korchak HM, Given WP, Abramson S, Weissmann G. Effects of non-steroidal anti-inflammatory agents on human neutrophil functions *in vitro* and *in vivo*. *Biochem Pharmacol* 1984; **33:** 371–8.
8. Kadurugamuwa JL, Hengstler B, Bray MA, Zak O. Inhibition of complement-factor-5A-induced inflammatory reactions by prostaglandin E_2 in experimental meningitis. *J Infect Dis* 1989; **160:** 715–19.

7
Prevention of Bacterial Meningitis

52. *The routine use of the* Haemophilus *b conjugate vaccines has significantly reduced the incidence of* Haemophilus influenzae *type b (Hib) meningitis*

Prior to the availability of effective vaccines, one in 200 children developed invasive *Haemophilus influenzae* type b (Hib) disease by the age of 5 years; 60% of these children had meningitis. Approximately two-thirds of all cases of Hib disease affect infants and children less than 15 months of age. Two Hib conjugate vaccines are currently licensed in the United States for administration to infants, from 2 months of age. These are the PRP–OMP vaccine and the HbOC vaccine. Antibody to the capsular polysaccharide of Hib (polyribosylribitolphosphate, PRP) plays a major role in host defense against this organism by promoting both opsonophagocytosis and bactericidal activity. Capsular polysaccharide itself is a poor immunogen in young infants because their B-lymphocytes respond poorly to polysaccharides.[1] Bacterial capsular polysaccharides are so-called T-cell-independent antigens, which have the following characteristics:

1. induction of a poor antibody response in infants and children younger than 18 months of age;
2. a quantitatively smaller antibody response than that seen with T-cell-dependent antigens;
3. an inability to induce a booster response.

Vaccines derived from the polyribosylribitolphosphate capsule of Hib were developed in the 1970s. These vaccines had an efficacy of 90% after one dose of vaccine in children 18–71 months old in a large trial in Finland. However, the vaccine was ineffective in infants 3–17 months of age.[2]

The immunogenicity of the vaccine is markedly improved by covalently linking the polysaccharide to a protein carrier (thus recruiting T-helper cells to enhance the immune response of B-cells) to produce a 'conjugate' vaccine. At the present time three different Hib conjugate vaccines are licensed for use in older children: HbOC, PRP–OMP and PRP-D. In the HbOC vaccine, the protein carrier is derived from a non-toxigenic mutant of diphtheria toxin covalently linked to several short oligosaccharides of PRP. In the PRP–OMP conjugate vaccine, outer-membrane proteins of *Neisseria meningitidis* (OMP) are linked to a medium-sized PRP polymer. The PRP-D vaccine consists of a medium-sized polysaccharide polymer linked to diphtheria toxoid.[3] Two of these three vaccines, HbOC and PRP–OMP, have been licensed for use in 2-month-olds. A level of 1.0 μg/mL of PRP antibody 1 month following vaccination (as measured by the Finnish Farr assay) appears to provide long-term protection against Hib.[1] Conjugate vaccines that contain either diphtheria toxoid or protein should not be considered as immunizing agents against diphtheria. Similarly, a conjugate vaccine that contains meningococcal protein should not be considered as an immunizing agent against meningococcal disease.[4]

The following recommendations for vaccine use are based on the Recommendations of the Immunization Practices Advisory Committee (1991)[4], and the Committee on Infectious Diseases of the American Academy of Pediatrics (1991)[5]:

1. All infants should be immunized with Hib conjugate vaccine (HbOC or PRP–OMP), starting at 2 months of age. Administration of the vaccine series may be initiated as early as 6 weeks of age. The Hib immunization can be given during visits currently scheduled for other routine immunizations, such as diphtheria–tetanus–pertussis, oral poliovirus and measles–mumps–rubella (MMR). The HbOC or PRP–OMP vaccine should be given intramuscularly at a separate site from other immunizations using a separate syringe.

2. Vaccine should not be interchanged once a dose has been started as the immunogenicity of HbOC and PRP–OMP are different, with the exception that any of the three licensed conjugate vaccines can be administered for the 15-month booster in the HbOC schedule.

3. If HbOC is to be used, previously unvaccinated infants 2–6 months of age should receive three doses given at least 2 months apart.
   (a) Unvaccinated infants 7–11 months of age should receive two doses of HbOC, given at least 2 months apart, before they are 15 months old.
   (b) Unvaccinated children 12–14 months of age should receive a single dose of vaccine before they are 15 months of age.
   (c) An additional dose of HbOC should be given to all children at 15 months of age, at an interval of not less than 2 months after the previous dose. The other two conjugate vaccines licensed for use at 15 months of age may be used for this dose, but there are no data demonstrating that a booster response will occur.

4. If PRP–OMP is to be used, previously unvaccinated infants 2–6 months of age should receive two doses 2 months apart and a booster dose at 12 months of age.
   (a) Children 7–11 months of age not previously vaccinated should receive two doses 2 months apart and a booster dose at 15 months of age, not less than 2 months after the previous dose.
   (b) Children 12–14 months of age not previously vaccinated should

   receive a single dose and a booster dose at 15 months of age. An interval as short as 1 month between doses is acceptable but not optimal.

5. At 15 months of age several immunizations are required, and more than one visit may be necessary to give these injections. Priority should be given to administering the MMR vaccine to children who have not been immunized previously against measles. *Haemophilus influenzae* type b conjugate vaccine and MMR vaccine can be administered simultaneously, but they should be administered at separate sites and with separate syringes.

6. Unvaccinated children 15–59 months of age may be given any of the three conjugate vaccines (HbOC, PRP–OMP, PRP–D) licensed for this age group. A single dose of any one of these licensed conjugate vaccines is recommended.

7. For infants born prematurely, immunization should be initiated at the chronologic age of 2 months as recommended for older infants (see recommendations 3 and 4).

8. Children younger than 24 months of age who have had invasive Hib disease should still be vaccinated, since many children in this age group fail to develop adequate immunity following natural disease.

9. Unvaccinated children 5 years of age or older with a chronic illness known to be associated with an increased risk of invasive Hib disease should be given a single dose of any licensed conjugate vaccine. Patients with Hodgkin's disease should be immunized 10–14 days or more prior to the initiation of chemotherapy or, if that is not possible, 3 months or more after the cessation of chemotherapy.

10. There are no known contraindications to simultaneous administration of any Hib conjugate vaccine with either the pneumococcal or meningococcal vaccines.

References

1. Kaplan SL. New aspects of prevention and therapy of meningitis. *Infect Dis Clin North Amer* 1992; **6**: 197–214.
2. Peltola H, Kayhty H, Sivonen A, Makela PH. *Haemophilus influenzae* type b capsular polysaccharide vaccine in children: a double-blind field study of 100,000 vaccinees 3 months to 5 years of age in Finland. *Pediatrics* 1977; **60**: 730–7.
3. Jones DM. Current and future trends in immunization against meningitis. *J Antimicrob Chemo* 1993; **31**(suppl B): 93–9.
4. Recommendations of the Immunization Practices Advisory Committee (ACIP). *Haemophilus* b conjugate vaccines for prevention of *Haemophilus influenzae* type b disease among infants and children two months of age and older. *MMWR* 1991; 40/No. RR-1:1–7.
5. Committee on Infectious Diseases American Academy of Pediatrics. *Haemophilus influenzae* type b conjugate vaccines: recommendations for immunization of infants and children 2 months of age and older. *Pediatrics* 1991; **88**: 169–72.

53.   *Serious adverse reactions to the Hib conjugate vaccines are rare, but there is an increased risk of Hib disease within several days of receiving the immunization*

The most common reactions to vaccination with the *Haemophilus influenzae* type b (Hib) conjugate vaccines are local reactions, such as redness, swelling and low-grade fever.[1] These reactions are more common following the third dose than after the first and second doses.

In a study of the safety and immunogenicity of the Hib–OMP vaccine in Apache and Navajo infants and children, 46 (13%) reactions related to the vaccine were reported in 348 vaccinations. None of these reactions were serious. Forty-five of the 46 reactions were localized swelling at the vaccination site. One child was irritable. Four children experienced a second reaction, in addition to localized swelling which included irritability, crying, fever and diarrhea. All of these symptoms resolved within 24 hours of onset.[2]

The safety and immunogenicity of a Hib conjugate (HbOC) vaccine was investigated in 103 infants in the United Kingdom immunized at 3, 5 and 9 months of age who also received diphtheria, pertussis and tetanus, and polio vaccines. Side effects were compared with 99 age-matched infants receiving diphtheria, pertussis and tetanus, and polio vaccines only. No major adverse reactions occurred in either group. Local reactions, defined as redness or swelling or warmth greater than 2 cm, occurred in 2% of infants after administration of the HbOC vaccine, and 19% of infants after the administration of the diphtheria, pertussis and tetanus vaccine.[3]

Three children (ages 19 months, 20 months and 33 months) developed an acute inflammatory demyelinating polyradiculoneuropathy (AIDP; Guillian–Barre syndrome) after immunization with the polyribosylribitolphosphate–diphtheria (PRP–D) conjugate vaccine. This vaccine consists of the polysaccharide polymer linked to diphtheria toxoid.[4] The onset of the AIDP occurred within 1 week of vaccination in all three children. Each received a different lot of the Hib PRP–D conjugate vaccine. One of the patients also received other vaccines (diphtheria–tetanus–pertussis and oral polio vaccines) that have anecdotally been associated with AIDP.

Invasive Hib infections have been observed in the week after immunization with capsular polysaccharide vaccine. The risk of depression of anticapsular antibody concentrations during the first week after immunization with Hib capsular polysaccharide–diphtheria conjugate vaccine was investigated in 30 infants, ages 18–21 months.[5] These investigators documented depression of antibody concentrations in 9 infants with pre-immunization anticapsular antibody concentrations (>0.025 μg/ml), and found that recovery of antibody concentrations occurred within 7 days of immunization. It appears, then, that a transient decline in PRP antibody may occur after the first PRP-D dose, if pre-existing antibody is circulating.[1] Whether or not this transient decline is associated with *H. influenzae* invasive disease is not known. There is a recovery in the anticapsular antibody concentration within one week of immunization.

References

1. Kaplan SL. New aspects of prevention and therapy in meningitis. *Infect Dis Clin North Amer* 1992; **6:** 197–214.
2. Santosham M, Hill J, Wolff M, et al. Safety and immunogenicity of a *Haemophilus influenzae* type b conjugate vaccine in a high risk American Indian population. *Pediatr Infect Dis J* 1991; **10:** 113–17.
3. Tudor-Williams G, Frankland J, Isaacs D, et al. *Haemophilus influenzae* type b conjugate vaccine trial in Oxford: implications for the United Kingdom. *Arch Dis Child* 1989; **64:** 520–4.
4. D'Cruz OF, Shapiro ED, Spiegelman KN, et al. Acute inflammatory demyelinating polyradiculoneuropathy (Guillain–Barre syndrome) after immunization with *Haemophilus influenzae* type b conjugate vaccine. *J Pediatr* 1989; **115:** 743–6.
5. Marchant CD, Band E, Froeschle JE, McVerry PH. Depression of anticapsular antibody after immunization with *Haemophilus influenzae* type b poly-saccharide–diphtheria conjugate vaccine. *Pediatr Infect Dis J* 1989; **8:** 508–11.

54.   In developed countries, routine vaccination with meningococcal vaccine is not recommended because the risk of infection is low and because the vaccine is not effective against serogroup B, which is responsible for the majority of meningococcal disease in these countries

Meningococcal vaccines have been important in controlling epidemics in Third World countries where group A meningococcal disease is constantly present with epidemics every few years. Immunity is, however, not long-lasting and is significantly reduced 3 to 5 years after vaccination.[1] The group A vaccine is efficacious in controlling local epidemics. Group C polysac-charide produces a weaker immune response than the group A poly-saccharide, and is poorly immunogenic in children under 2 years of age. The group C meningococcal vaccine has been used effectively in outbreaks of meningitis, particularly in schools and military camps, where lasting protection is not required.[2,3] Immunoprophylaxis of meningococcal disease currently uses a quadrivalent (serogroups A, C, Y and W135) polysaccharide vaccine. Only the group A meningococcal vaccine component of the quadrivalent capsular polysaccharide vaccine provides protective antibody in infants.[4] Vaccination is recommended only for high-risk individuals, including travelers to countries with hyperendemic or epidemic disease, in outbreaks due to those serogroups in the vaccine, for individuals in the military, and for persons at high risk, such as those individuals with terminal-complement-component deficiencies and for individuals who have had a splenectomy.[5]

Serogroup B is responsible for the majority of meningococcal disease in developed countries. The polysaccharide capsule of this organism is poorly immunogenic because anti-B polysaccharide antibodies are not bactericidal in the presence of human complement.[2,6] In order to improve the immunogenicity of the serogroup B polysaccharide, a polysaccharide–protein conjugate vaccine, similar to the *Haemophilus influenzae* type b conjugate vaccine, has been developed. Vaccines composed of outer-membrane proteins from serotypes 2b and 15 (which together are responsible for most outbreaks of group B disease) noncovalently complexed to serogroup B capsular polysaccharide have been demonstrated to induce bactericidal antibodies in adult volunteers.[5,7]

References

1. Reingold AL, Broome CV, Hightower AW, et al. Age-specific differences in duration of clinical protection after vaccination with meningococcal polysaccharide A vaccine. *Lancet* 1985; **ii:** 114–18.
2. Jones DM. Current and future trends in immunization against meningitis. *J Antimicrob Chemo* 1993; **31**(suppl B): 93–9.
3. Masterton RG, Youngs ER, Wardle KR, et al. Epidemiology-control of an outbreak of group C meningococcal meningitis with a polysaccharide vaccine. *J Infect* 1988; **17:** 177–82.
4. Feigin RD, McCracken GH, Klein JO. Diagnosis and management of meningitis. *Pediatr Infect Dis J* 1992; **11:** 785–814.
5. Swartz M. Acute bacterial meningitis. In: Gorbach SL, Bartlett JG, Blacklow NR (eds), *Infectious Diseases*. Philadelphia: W.B. Saunders, 1992; 1160–77.
6. Skevakis L, Frasch CE, Zahradnik JM, Dolin R. Class-specific human bactericidal antibodies to capsular and noncapsular surface antigens of *Neisseria meningitidis*. *J Infect Dis* 1984; **149:** 387–96.
7. Frasch CE, Zahradnick JM, Wang LY, Mocca LF, Tsai C-M. Antibody response of adults to an aluminum hydroxide-absorbed *Neisseria meningitidis* serotype 2b protein-group B polysaccharide vaccine. *J Infect Dis* 1988; **158:** 710–18.

55.   *The pneumococcal vaccine is not yet suitable for the prevention of meningitis in children younger than 5 years of age*

As the incidence of *Haemophilus influenzae* type b (Hib) meningitis decreases due to the routine use of the Hib conjugate vaccines, the incidence of pneumococcal meningitis is expected to increase. The current pneumococcal vaccines consist of a mixture of capsular polysaccharides derived from up to 23 serotypes.[1] Although immunogenic and protective in adults, when young children are vaccinated they are unable to produce a significant increase in antibody to the specific serotype for which protection is most desirable. This poor response occurs in children up to 5 years of age at least and perhaps older. In a controlled double-blind efficacy trial of a 14-valent pneumococcal vaccine, serum samples were analyzed by radioimmunoassay for type-specific pneumococcal antibody in 249 children aged 6–54 months.[2] Levels of serum antibody to all serotypes increased after immunization in all age groups tested. Responses were poor up to the age of 5 years for the important pediatric serotypes (6A, 14, 19F, and 23F). Seventeen children under the age of 2 years at the time of primary immunization received booster doses of vaccine 6 months later. There was no significant increase in antibody to any serotype, and the geometric mean antibody levels fell for most types. Immune response to the pediatric serotypes was poor until the age of 4.5 years.

The current pneumococcal polysaccharide vaccine is only 60–70% effective in adults.[3] It is ineffective in children less than 2 years of age. The Immunization Practices Advisory Committee of the Public Health Service[4] recommends the immunization of individuals who are 65 years of age and older, and others at risk, including adults and children with chronic disease, such as diabetes, congestive heart failure, pulmonary disease, hepatic or renal disease, and immunocompromised persons, such as those infected with the human immunodeficiency virus, individuals with multiple myeloma or an asplenic state, and those with cancer. Individuals with a CSF fistula or leak should also be vaccinated. The dose of the vaccine is 0.5 mL intramuscularly. Booster injections should be given every 5 years. The decision whether to administer these vaccines to children between the ages of 2 and 5 years must be individualized.

Preliminary results of studies with a new conjugate pneumococcal vaccine suggests that this vaccine is immunogenic in infants and young children. However, it is not known whether this vaccine will affect colonization or prevent disease on the basis of serotypes contained in the vaccine.[5]

References

1. Jones DM. Current and future trends in immunization against meningitis. *J Antimicrob Chemo* 1993; **31** (suppl B): 93–9.
2. Douglas RM, Paton JC, Duncan SJ, Hansman DJ. Antibody response to pneumococcal vaccination in children younger than five years of age. *J Infect Dis* 1983; **148:** 131–7.
3. Bolan G, Broome CV, Facklam RR, et al. Pneumococcal vaccine efficacy in selected populations in the United States. *Ann Intern Med* 1986; **104:** 1–6.
4. Recommendations of the Immunization Practices Advisory Committee: pneumococcal polysaccharide vaccine. *MMWR Morb Mortal Wkly Rep* 1989; **38:** 64–8, 73–6.
5. Friedland IR, McCracken GH. To the Editor. *N Engl J Med* 1994; **331:** 1775.

56.   *Rifampin is the currently recommended antibiotic for prophylaxis of meningococcal meningitis*

Chemoprophylaxis is used for the prevention of secondary cases once an index case has been identified. The risk of meningitis in household contacts of an index case is approximately 4 in 1,000, which is 500-fold to 1,000-fold greater than for the general population, and is particularly increased in young children.[1] The risk of developing secondary meningitis is highest immediately after contact with an index case, with the majority of secondary cases occurring within the first week after the index case. The risk of meningitis remains higher in family households for a prolonged period of time, and secondary cases have been reported as late as 2 months after the index case.[2]

Asymptomatic nasopharyngeal carriage of meningococci is common in healthy individuals, and carriage rates can vary from 1% to 35% during a single year.[3] During one outbreak of *Neisseria meningitidis* meningitis, students in the same classroom as the index case had higher carriage rates than the students in other classrooms in the same school, but the risk of developing meningitis was not increased. The cases of meningitis that occurred among household contacts of the index case were more likely to have had close contact with other students in the school than controls, suggesting the possibility that school children bring the infection to their family members at home through asymptomatic carriage.[2,4]

The transmission of meningococci is facilitated by crowding (army barracks, boarding schools and prisons), close contact, low socio-economic conditions, low humidity, concomitant viral infections (especially respiratory viruses) and smoking. At least three host factors are important in determining whether a newly infected individual will become an asymptomatic carrier or develop meningitis:

1. the presence of specific functional antibodies (for opsonophagocytosis and bactericidal activity);
2. an intact complement pathway (individuals with terminal complement component deficiencies are more susceptible to fulminant meningococcal disease);
3. a normal reticuloendothelial system.[2]

Close contacts of the index case should receive chemoprophylaxis as soon as the primary case is identified. Close contacts are defined as household, daycare and nursery school individuals who have had contact with the patient's oral secretions and medical personnel performing mouth-to-mouth resuscitation without precautionary equipment.

During World War II, sulfonamides were used to provide prophylaxis.[5] Oral sulfadiazine at a dose of 1.0 g every 12 hours for a 2-day course in adults was very effective in eradicating carriage of susceptible strains. Widespread sulfonamide resistance was first recognized in 1963, but has declined since then. For this reason, sulfonamides should not be used for prophylaxis unless the sensitivity of the meningococci has been established.[2] Sulfisoxazole is recommended when an isolate is known to be susceptible – a 2-day course of 500 mg daily for infants younger than 1 year, 500 mg every 12 hours for children 1–12 years, and 1 g every 12 hours for children older than 12 years and adults.[6] Rifampin is currently the recommended antimicrobial agent for chemoprophylaxis. The recommended dose is 600 mg every 12 hours for 2 days in adults, 10 mg/kg every 12 hours for 2 days in children older than 1 year of age, and 5 mg/kg every 12 hours for 2 days in children younger than 1 year of age. As rifampin-resistant meningococci have been reported where mass prophylaxis has been used,[7] the sensitivity of the meningococci to the chosen agent for prophylaxis should be monitored. Rifampin should not be used during pregnancy.

A single intramuscular injection of ceftriaxone (250 mg) was effective in eradicating meningococcal carriage in family contacts during an outbreak of group A meningococcal meningitis in Saudi Arabia.[8]

Ciprofloxacin administered in a single dose has been 93–97% effective in eradicating meningococci from the nasopharynx.[9,10] Ciprofloxacin has the advantage of being effective after a single oral dose. There is some concern about using ciprofloxacin in individuals less than 18 years of age because of the risk of arthropathy. Ciprofloxacin accumulates in bone when given in large doses in experimental studies. It is unlikely that a single dose would have any adverse effect on bone development, and therefore a single dose is probably safe in children. Table 56.1 lists the recommended dosages of the various antibiotics for the chemoprophylaxis of meningococcal meningitis.

Table 56.1 Chemoprophylaxis of meningococcal meningitis

Antibiotic	Dose
Rifampin (oral agent)	Adults: 600 mg every 12 h for 2 days Children (>1 year): 10 mg/kg every 12 h for 2 days Children (<1 year): 5 mg/kg every 12 h for 2 days
Ceftriaxone (intramuscular injection)	Adults: 250 mg Children: 125 mg
Ciprofloxacin (oral agent)	Single dose – 750 mg
Sulfisoxazole (oral agent)	Adults: 1 g every 12 h for 2 days Children (1–12 years): 500 mg every 12 h for 2 days Children (<1 year): 500 mg daily for 2 days

Source: Feigin (1992).[6]

Chemoprophylaxis should be given to the index patient prior to hospital discharge. During an epidemic, vaccination is recommended, as individuals are liable to become reinfected soon after prophylaxis.

References

1. Meningococcal Disease Surveillance Group. Meningococcal disease: secondary attack rate and chemoprophylaxis in the United States, 1974. *JAMA* 1976; **235:** 261–5.
2. Cuevas LE, Hart CA. Chemoprophylaxis of bacterial meningitis. *J Antimicrob Chemo* 1993; **31**(suppl B): 79–91.
3. Ichhpujani RL, Mohan R, Grover SS, Joshi PR, Kumari S. Nasopharyngeal carriage of *Neisseria meningitidis* in the general population and meningococcal disease. *J Comm Dis* 1990; **22:** 264–8.
4. Hudson PJ, Vogt RL, Heun EM, Brondum J, et al. Evidence for school transmission of *Neisseria meningitidis* during a Vermont outbreak. *Pediatr Infect Dis* 1986; **5:** 213–17.
5. Kuhns DM, Nelson CT, Feldman HA, Kuhn LR. The prophylactic value of sulfadiazine in the control of meningococcic meningitis. *JAMA* 1943; **123:** 335–9.
6. Feigin RD, McCracken GH, Klein J. Diagnosis and management of meningitis. *Pediatr Infect Dis J* 1992; **11:** 785–814.
7. Schubiger G, Munzinger J, Dudli C, Wipfli U. Meningokokken-epidemic in einer internatsschule: sekundarerkrangkung mit rifampicin – resistantem erreger unter chemoprophylaxe. *Schweiz Med Wochenschr* 1986; **116:** 1172–5.
8. Schwartz B, Al-Tobaiqi A, Al-Puwais A, Fontane RE, et al. Comparative efficacy of ceftriaxone and rifampicin in eradicating pharyngeal carriage of group A *Neisseria meningitidis*. *Lancet* 1988; **i:** 1239–42.
9. Pugsley MP, Dworzack DL, Horowitz EA, Cuevas TA, et al. Efficacy of ciprofloxacin in the treatment of nasopharyngeal carriers of *Neisseria meningitidis*. *J Infect Dis* 1987; **156:** 211–13.
10. Gaunt PN, Lambert BE. Single dose ciprofloxacin for the eradication of pharyngeal carriage of *Neisseria meningitidis*. *J Antimicrob Chemo* 1988; **21:** 489–96.

57.   A 4-day course of rifampin is recommended for prophylaxis of Hib meningitis, not a 2-day course of therapy, as recommended for prophylaxis of meningococcal meningitis

The risk of secondary disease from close contact with an individual with *Haemophilus influenzae* type b (Hib) meningitis is age-dependent, being highest for children less than 2 years of age. Epidemics of *H.. influenzae* meningitis do not occur, although clustering of cases does occur.[1] The nasopharyngeal carrier rate for Hib is usually less than 5%, but colonization is also age-dependent with the highest rates found among the youngest siblings of a patient. Once Hib colonizes the nasopharynx, it can be recovered for periods of up to 1 year, suggesting that prolonged carriage is not unusual.[1,2]

The spread of virulent strains of Hib has been of particular concern in daycare centers in industrialized countries. The risk of secondary disease for children 0–23 months of age that share the same classroom with the index case appears to be a risk similar to that reported for household contacts.[3]

Chemoprophylaxis does not eradicate the organism from the upper respiratory tract, therefore the index patient should receive chemoprophylaxis before discharge from the hospital, especially if there will be exposure to household members who are younger than 4 years of age. Prophylaxis is recommended for all members of a household if there is a child in the household that is younger than 48 months.

The American Academy of Pediatrics recommends rifampin prophylaxis (20 mg/kg/day orally for 4 days – maximum 600 mg/day) for all individuals in households with at least one child younger than 24 months or with a non-immunized child 24–48 months of age.[4] Prophylaxis for children in daycare centers should be provided if the center resembles a household environment with children under 2 years of age attending for prolonged periods of more than 25 hours per week. All the members of the staff and school attendees of the center should receive prophylaxis. In addition, prophylaxis is recommended for any daycare center where a second case of Hib meningitis occurs within 60 days.[1] Pregnant women should not be given rifampin.

References

1. Cuevas LE, Hart CA. Chemoprophylaxis of bacterial meningitis. *J Antimicrob Chemo* 1993; **31**(suppl B): 79–91.
2. Ginsburg CM, McCracken GH, Rae S, Parke JC. *Haemophilus influenzae* type b disease. Incidence in a day care center. *JAMA* 1977; **238**: 604–7.
3. Flemming DW, Leibenhaut MH, Albanes D, Cochi SL, et al. Secondary *Haemophilus influenzae* type b in day-care facilities. *JAMA* 1985; **254**: 509–14.
4. Committee on Infectious Diseases. Revision of recommendation for use of rifampin prophylaxis of contacts of patients with *Haemophilus influenzae* infection. *Pediatrics* 1984; **74**: 301–2.

8
Aseptic Meningitis

58. *Aseptic meningitis is, by definition, a disease with the clinical presentation of meningitis, mild CSF abnormalities and a fairly benign course*

Viral meningitis and aseptic meningitis are terms which are used interchangeably but probably should not be. The defining criteria of aseptic meningitis were described by Wallgren in 1925 and are as follows:

1. acute onset;
2. meningeal signs and symptoms;
3. CSF abnormalities typical of meningitis with a predominance of mononuclear cells;
4. absence of bacteria on smear and by culture of CSF;
5. no parameningeal focus of infection;
6. self-limited benign course.[1-3]

The classic CSF abnormalities are a mononuclear or lymphocytic pleocytosis with the absence of bacteria. The differential diagnosis of a CSF lymphocytic pleocytosis is much broader than one disease entity (i.e. viral meningitis) and includes infectious and non-infectious etiologies (Tables 58.1 and 58.2). The differential diagnosis of acute aseptic meningitis is also the differential diagnosis of viral meningitis.

In performing CSF examinations on patients with a clinical presentation suggestive of viral meningitis it is useful to send CSF to the laboratory for routine studies (Table 58.3) and to save a small amount of CSF until the cell count and glucose concentration are known. This practice avoids getting the result "quantity not sufficient" for the key diagnostic test on CSF in the patient where CSF was obtained with great difficulty. Alternatively, repeat lumbar puncture can be performed and any diagnostic studies not obtained on the initial CSF examination can be obtained on the subsequent examination. Repeat CSF examination will most likely be necessary in any patient who has persistent symptoms for a duration longer than 10 days.

Table 58.1   Differential diagnosis of cerebrospinal fluid lymphocytic pleocytosis infectious etiologies

Viral
Enteroviruses
Mumps
Lymphocytic choriomeningitis (LCM) virus
Herpes simplex virus (HSV)
Human immunodeficiency virus (HIV)
Arthropod-borne viruses

Non-viral
Mycobacterium tuberculosis
Listeria monocytogenes
Mycoplasma pneumoniae
Rickettsia rickettsii (Rocky Mountain spotted fever)
Treponema pallidum (syphilis)
Borrelia burgdorferi (Lyme disease)
Cryptococcus neoformans, Coccidioides immites,
    Histoplasma capsulatum

Other
Partially treated bacterial meningitis
Parameningeal focus of infection
Meningitis complicating endocarditis
Parainfectious syndrome (acute disseminated
    encephalomyelitis)

Table 58.2   Differential diagnosis of cerebrospinal fluid lymphocytic pleocytosis non-infectious etiologies

Systemic lupus erythematosus
Sarcoidosis
Migraine
Traumatic lumbar puncture
Chronic benign lymphocytic meningitis
Vasculitis
Meningeal carcinomatosis
Medications (ibuprofen, isoniazid, azathioprine,
    trimethoprim (± sulfonamides), OKT3, sulindac,
    tolmetin, naproxen)

Source: Connolly and Hammer (1990);[1] Wilhelm (1992).

In addition to a neurologic examination, a neuroimaging study and a CSF examination, all patients should have a chest X-ray, blood, urine, throat and stool cultures, and HIV and syphilis serology.

Table 58.3   Routine studies on cerebrospinal fluid

Opening pressure
Cell count
Chemistries
Venereal disease research laboratory test (VDRL)
Bacterial smear and culture
Viral culture
India ink, fungal culture
Cryptococcal antigen
Acid-fast bacilli smear and culture

Table 58.4 provides specific laboratory tests to diagnose specific disease entities.

Table 58.4   Laboratory tests to diagnose etiology of cerebrospinal fluid lymphocytic pleocytosis

Infectious agent	Laboratory test
Enterovirus	CSF viral culture Throat washing Stool culture Serum for acute and convalescent IgG antibody
Arthropod-borne viruses	CSF or blood viral culture
Herpes simplex virus type 2	CSF viral culture Serum for acute and convalescent IgG antibody Genital lesions
HIV	HIV blood serology; if negative, repeat in 3–6 months
Lymphocytic choriomeningitis virus	CSF viral culture Blood viral culture Serum for acute and convalescent IgG antibody
Mumps virus	CSF viral culture
Treponema pallidum	Serum and CSF VDRL Serum FTA
Borrelia burgdorferi	Lyme serology CSF Lyme antibody index
Mycoplasma pneumoniae	Serum cold agglutinins
Mycobacterium tuberculosis	PPD CSF smear for acid-fast bacilli CSF culture CSF tuberculostearic acid assay

Table 58.4   Laboratory tests to diagnose etiology of cerebrospinal fluid (CSF) lymphocytic pleocytosis *continued*

Infectious agent	Laboratory test
Sarcoidosis	Angiotensin converting enzyme Chest X-ray (hilar adenopathy) Conjunctival, lymph node or salivary gland biopsy
Cryptococcus neoformans	India ink smear and culture Cryptococcal antigen (CSF)
Coccidioides immites	India ink smear and culture
Histoplasma capsulatum	India ink smear and culture *Histoplasma* polysaccharide antigen (CSF)
Vasculitis	Angiography Leptomeningeal or brain biopsy

HIV, human immunodeficiency virus; VDRL, venereal disease research laboratory; FTA, fluorescent treponemal antibody; PPD, purified protein derivative.

References

1. Connolly KJ, Hammer SM. The acute aseptic meningitis syndrome. *Infect Dis Clin North Amer* 1990; **4**: 599–622.
2. Adair CV, Gauld RL, Smadel JE. Aseptic meningitis, a disease of diverse etiology: clinical and etiologic studies on 854 cases. *Ann Intern Med* 1953; **39**: 675–704.
3. Wallgren A. Une nouvelle maladie infectieuse du systeme nerveux central: (Meningite aseptique aique). *Acta Paediatr* 1925; **4**: 158–82.

59.   *The level of consciousness is normal in viral meningitis*

Individuals with viral meningitis appear acutely ill, complain of frontal or retro-orbital headache, photophobia, myalgias, and nausea and vomiting but are typically awake and alert.[1] The most striking complaint is that of a severe "grippe-like" headache. On examination, there is evidence of meningeal irritation and the patient may be lethargic, but patients with viral meningitis are not obtunded or comatose. The presence of focal neurologic deficits is typical of viral encephalitis, specifically herpes simplex virus encephalitis, and should be treated as such. Focal neurologic deficits do not occur in a benign self-limited viral meningitis. Enterovirus infections may be associated with a maculopapular, vesicular or petechial systemic rash.[2] There may be evidence of genital vesicular lesions or a history of recurrent genital herpes in herpes simplex virus type 2 meningitis.

References

1. Bale JF. Meningitis and encephalitis. In: McKendall RR, Stroop WG (eds), *Handbook of Neurovirology*. New York: Marcel Dekker, 1994, 141–58.
2. Rubeiz H, Roos RP. Viral meningitis and encephalitis. *Semin Neurol* 1992; **12:** 165–77.

60. *Enteroviruses are the most common infectious agents of viral meningitis for which an etiology can be determined*

The enteroviruses are a family of viruses that include poliovirus, Coxsackieviruses A and B, echoviruses and the newer enteroviruses 68–71 and 72 (hepatitis A).[1] The serotypes most often responsible for viral meningitis are echovirus types 6, 9 and 20 and Coxsackieviruses A9, B2, B3 and B5.[2] There is also a seasonal variation to viruses causing meningitis, with enteroviruses and arthropod-borne viruses predominating in the summer and early autumn and lymphocytic choriomeningitis (LCM) virus being more prevalent in the fall and winter.[2]

Enteroviruses inhabit the alimentary tract and are spread from host to host by the fecal–hand–oral route of transmission. Enterovirus infections peak in summer and early fall. The clinical presentation of enterovirus meningitis includes headache, fever, pharyngitis, lethargy, nausea, vomiting and meningismus. The CSF has a mild pleocytosis with a white blood cell (WBC) count usually less than 1000/mm³ and a predominance of lymphocytes (although initially there may be a predominance of polymorphonuclear leukocytes). The protein concentration may be mildly elevated; the glucose concentration is usually normal.[1] The CSF, stool and oropharynx should be cultured for virus. The stool is the most likely source for virus isolation.[2] If enterovirus is isolated from a non-CSF viral culture, a presumptive diagnosis of enteroviral meningitis can be made. A definitive diagnosis of enteroviral meningitis requires a positive CSF viral culture[3] or a four-fold rise in serum virus antibody. Acute and convalescent serum samples should be obtained for antibody titers. The virus causing infection can be identified by detecting a four-fold or greater increase in antiviral IgG antibody, or the first-time appearance of virus-specific IgM antibodies.[4] The detection of intrathecally synthesized enterovirus-specific antibodies (virus-specific oligoclonal antibodies) in CSF is useful in the diagnosis of enterovirus infection of the CNS.[5] This laboratory investigation would require sending CSF to the laboratory with a request for isoelectric focusing and affinity-mediated immunoblot identification of enterovirus-specific oligoclonal antibodies.

Polymerase chain reaction tests to enable rapid detection of virus nucleic acid in CSF are being developed. Each virus has its own specific nucleic acid sequence. The currently available deoxyribonucleic acid (DNA) probe techniques (which use a nucleic acid sequence that binds to a genetic sequence in the virus) are not sensitive enough to detect the small amount of viral DNA in infected CSF.[6] The polymerase chain reaction amplifies minute amounts of nucleic acid sequences allowing for the rapid identification of the infecting virus within 24 to 48 hours.

Enterovirus meningitis is typically self-limiting and treatment is supportive.

References

1. Connolly KJ, Hammer SM. The acute aseptic meningitis syndrome. *Infect Dis Clin North Amer* 1990; **4:** 599–622.
2. Rubeiz H, Roos RP. Viral meningitis and encephalitis. *Semin Neurol* 1992; **12:** 165–77.
3. Johnson GM, McAbee GA, Seaton ED, Lipson SM. Suspect value of non-CSF viral cultures in the diagnosis of enteroviral CNS infection in young infants. *Dev Med Child Neurol* 1992; **34:** 876–84.
4. Bale JF. Meningitis and encephalitis. In: McKendall RR, Stroop WG (eds), *Handbook of Neurovirology*. New York: Marcel Dekker, 1994; 141–58.
5. Kaiser R, Dorries R, Martin R, Fuhrmeister U, Leonhardt KF, ter Meulen V. Intrathecal synthesis of virus-specific oligoclonal antibodies in patients with enterovirus infection of the central nervous system. *J Neurol* 1989; **236:** 395–9.
6. Overall JC. Is it bacterial or viral; laboratory differentiation. *Pediatr Rev* 1993; **14:** 251–61.

61.   *Herpes simplex virus type 2 causes an aseptic meningitis*

Herpes simplex virus type 2 (HSV-2) causes genital disease and aseptic meningitis. In a series of 182 cases of primary genital HSV-2 infection in women, 36% had aseptic meningitis. Among 104 men with primary genital HSV-2 infection, 13% had aseptic meningitis.[1] The meningitis usually occurs during a primary genital infection; however, meningitis may occur with recurrence of genital lesions and HSV-2 may be isolated from the CSF in the absence of genital lesions.[1,2]

The diagnosis of HSV-2 aseptic meningitis may be suggested clinically by identification of genital vesicular lesions or complaints of urinary retention or radicular symptoms, in association with headache, fever and mild photophobia. Cerebrospinal fluid examination typically demonstrates a lymphocytic pleocytosis (300–400 cells/mm^3) with an elevated protein concentration. The glucose concentration may be normal or decreased.[3] A definitive diagnosis requires either a positive CSF viral culture or demonstration of a four-fold rise in HSV-2-specific IgG. The meningitis is typically self-limiting. Antiviral therapy is, however, recommended for meningitis that occurs in association with a primary genital herpes infection.[2]

Intravenous acyclovir therapy is a slightly more effective treatment for a primary genital herpes infection than oral acyclovir therapy. The recommended dosage is 5 mg/kg intravenously every 8 hours for 5 days.[4]

Oral acyclovir therapy is almost as effective as intravenous therapy for the initial episode of genital herpes and can be recommended in otherwise healthy individuals. Treatment is generally indicated for primary genital herpes infections; when this is associated with aseptic meningitis, hospitalization and intravenous antiviral therapy are recommended.[5]

References

1. Corey L, Adams HG, Brown ZA, Holmes KK. Genital herpes simplex virus infections: clinical manifestations, course and complications. *Ann Intern Med* 1983; **98:** 958–72.
2. Rubeiz H, Roos RP. Viral meningitis and encephalitis. *Semin Neurol* 1992; **12:** 165–77.
3. Brenton DW. Hypoglycorrhachia in herpes simplex type 2 meningitis. *Arch Neurol* 1980; **37:** 317.
4. Whitley RJ, Gnann JW. Acyclovir: a decade later. *N Engl J Med* 1992; **11:** 782–9.
5. Connolly KJ, Hammer SM. The acute aseptic meningitis syndrome. *Infect Dis Clin North Amer* 1990; **4:** 599–622.

62.   Human immunodeficiency virus (HIV) infection may cause meningitis prior to detection of a positive serology

Within 3 to 6 weeks of initial infection, the human immunodeficiency virus (HIV) may cause a mononucleosis-like syndrome with fever, generalized lymphadenopathy, pharyngeal infection, rash, malaise, myalgias, arthralgias and splenomegaly. An aseptic meningitis syndrome may develop during this acute illness characterized by headache, stiff neck, photophobia and encephalopathy. Human immunodeficiency virus serology may not yet be reactive and, if initially negative, should be repeated in 3 to 6 months in individuals at risk of HIV infection. Cerebrospinal fluid examination reveals an increased protein (< 100 mg/dL), mononuclear pleocytosis (< 200 cells/mm^3) and a normal or slightly decreased glucose concentration. Human immunodeficiency virus may be cultured from CSF but the overall isolation rate is not known.[1-3] Human immunodeficiency virus 1 aseptic meningitis is self-limited, but may take up to 4 weeks to resolve.

Cerebrospinal fluid abnormalities, specifically a sterile pleocytosis, are very common on routine examination of the CSF in asymptomatic HIV-infected individuals without clinically detectable neurologic disease.[1,4] Cerebrospinal fluid examinations were performed on 459 asymptomatic, neurologically normal, HIV-positive individuals. There was at least one abnormality in 60% of the CSF samples from these individuals: 6.4 % had an elevated protein concentration, 15.6% had nucleated cell counts greater than 10/mm^3, 14% had oligoclonal bands, 10% had an IgG synthesis rate of greater than 15 mg/dL (about 4.5 times the upper limit of normal), 11.6% had an elevated IgG index, and 10% had an elevated CSF IgG concentration. These CSF abnormalities were not, however, predictive of the subsequent development of neurologic disease. In this same series, there was also a decline in the CSF glucose concentration and in the degree of CSF pleocytosis between the group of patients who were HIV-positive only and the groups of patients with HIV-positivity and decreased T-helper cells and/or opportunistic infections. The decline in the CSF glucose concentration between the groups was attributed to the metabolic effects of a chronic CNS viral infection. The decline in the degree of CSF pleocytosis between the groups was attributed to an inability to mount a cellular response in the CSF reflecting the impaired cellular response characteristic of the peripheral immune system late in the disease. Overall, patients with HIV and or decreased T-helper cells and/or opportunistic infections had fewer CSF abnormalities than patients with HIV-positivity only.[4]

References

1. Berger JR, Levy RM. The neurologic complications of human immunodeficiency virus infection. *Med Clin North Amer* 1993; **77**: 1–23.
2. Connolly KJ, Hammer SM. The acute aseptic meningitis syndrome. *Infect Dis Clin North Amer* 1990; **4**: 599–622.
3. Hollander H, Stringau S. Human immunodeficiency virus-associated meningitis. Clinical course and correlations. *Am J Med* 1987; **83**: 813–86.
4. Marshall DW, Brey RL, Cahill WT, et al. Spectrum of cerebrospinal fluid findings in various stages of human immunodeficiency virus infection. *Arch Neurol* 1988; **45**: 954–8.

63.   *Mumps virus and lymphocytic choriomeningitis virus are two of the few viral etiologies of aseptic meningitis with a decreased CSF glucose*

The most common neurologic complication of mumps and the mumps vaccine is an aseptic meningitis. Both mumps virus and the vaccine strain mumps virus can cause meningitis. In both cases, the incubation period is about 21 days. Since the introduction of the mumps vaccine in the USA in 1967, there has been a marked decline in the incidence of mumps. The mumps vaccine contains a live attenuated mumps virus. The most common neurologic complication of mumps and of the mumps immunization is meningitis. This is a much more benign illness than meningoencephalitis complicating natural mumps.[1] Vaccine-related mumps meningitis has been reported in Canada, the United Kingdom and Japan and has been associated with the measles–mumps–rubella vaccine containing the Urabe AM-9 mumps virus. In the United States, the Jeryl–Lynn mumps virus is used in the vaccine and cases of aseptic meningitis have not been reported.[2]

Mumps and mumps-vaccine meningitis present with fever, headache and vomiting. Mumps encephalitis presents with fever, altered consciousness, seizures and focal neurologic deficits. The incidence of encephalitis within 30 days of immunization with the mumps vaccine in the United States is 0.4 per one million doses.[3] The typical CSF abnormalities in mumps meningitis are as follows:

1. normal opening pressure;
2. white blood cell count of 300–600 cells/mm^3, with a lymphocytic predominance, although polymorphonuclear leukocytes may predominate in the early stages of infection;
3. normal or slightly elevated protein concentration;
4. the glucose concentration is normal in the majority of cases, but glucose concentrations of 20–40 mg/dL may be present in 10–20% of cases.[2,4]

Cerebrospinal fluid viral culture is required for definitive diagnosis. The serologic tests are not useful in patients who have recently been immunized as a four-fold rise in mumps-specific IgG may simply represent successful immunization. Mumps meningitis is a self-limiting illness with a complete recovery.

The lymphocytic choriomeningitis (LCM) virus can cause human disease following contact with infected mice and hamsters. Meningeal symptoms are often preceded by a flu-like illness with fever, malaise, myalgias and arthralgias and occasionally alopecia.[5] The clinical presentation of meningitis is typical of viral meningitis with fever, headache, stiff neck, nausea and vomiting. Cerebrospinal fluid examination demonstrates a lymphocytic pleocytosis and a decreased glucose concentration. Diagnosis is made by culturing virus from blood or CSF or by demonstrating a four-fold rise in virus-specific antibodies. Meningitis due to the LCM virus is typically a self-limited disease; however, if the infection is acquired during pregnancy there is a risk of either spontaneous abortion or congenital malformations – hydrocephalus and chorioretinitis.[6]

References

1. Anonymous. Mumps meningitis and MMR vaccination. *Lancet* 1989; ii(8670): 1015–16.
2. Gnann JW. Mumps virus diseases. In: McKendall RR, Stroop WG (eds), *Handbook of Neurovirology*. New York: Marcel Dekker, 1994; 563–73.
3. Anonymous. Mumps prevention. Recommendations of the Immunization Practices Advisory Committee (ACIP). *MMWR* 1989; **38:** 388–400.
4. Johnstone JA, Ross CAC, Dunn M. Meningitis and encephalitis associated with mumps infection. *Arch Dis Child* 1972; **47:** 647–51.
5. Rubeiz H, Roos RP. Viral meningitis and encephalitis. *Semin Neurol* 1992; **12:** 165–77.

6. Lehmann-Grube F. Diseases of the nervous system caused by lymphocytic choriomeningitis virus and other arenaviruses. In: Vinken PJ, Bruyn GW, Klawans HL, McKendall RR (eds), *Handbook of Clinical Neurology*. New York: Elsevier Science Publishers, 1989; 355–81.

64.   *There are several CSF markers that are helpful in distinguishing viral from bacterial meningitis*

There is typically a CSF pleocytosis with a predominance of lymphocytes in viral meningitis, but early on there may be a predominance of polymorphonuclear leukocytes (PMNs). When the latter is detected, a repeat CSF examination 12 hours later should reveal the characteristic lymphocytic predominance.[1] It is possible, however, that a second lumbar puncture will not show a shift from a polymorphonuclear leukocyte to a lymphocyte predominance. When this occurs, the decision whether or not to treat the patient with antibiotics should be based on the clinical course and the results of CSF Gram's stain and culture.[2]

A CSF lactate acid concentration of >35 mg/dL is suggestive of bacterial meningitis. The CSF lactic acid concentration is typically <35 mg/dL in viral meningitis.[3,4]

Several studies have demonstrated an elevation in the concentration of tumor necrosis factor-alpha (TNF-alpha) in CSF from children and adults with acute bacterial meningitis, but not in cases of enteroviral meningitis.[5-9] In one study, elevated concentrations of TNF-alpha were observed in 42 of 51 patients with bacterial meningitis and in only 5 of 78 patients with nonbacterial meningitis. Normal concentrations of TNF-alpha were observed in CSF in all 44 patients with meningitis caused by enteroviruses. The 5 patients who had a moderate elevation in the concentration of TNF-alpha with nonbacterial meningitis had either herpes simplex virus type 2 or varicella-zoster virus encephalitis.[9] The earlier that CSF is sampled in the course of bacterial meningitis, the higher or more abnormal the CSF TNF-alpha concentration will be.

Elevated CSF interferon and interleukin-1 beta concentrations have been reported in viral meningitis and herpes simplex virus encephalitis, and therefore cannot be used to distinguish viral from bacterial meningitis.[10-13]

References

1. Dalton M, Newton RW. Aseptic meningitis. *Dev Med Child Neurol* 1991; **33**: 446–58.
2. Harrison SA, Risser WL. Repeat lumbar puncture in the differential diagnosis of meningitis. *Pediatr Infect Dis J* 1988; **7**: 143–5.
3. Brook I, Bricknell KS, Overturf GD, Finegold SM. Measurement of lactic acid in

cerebrospinal fluid of patients with infections of the central nervous system. *J Infect Dis* 1978; **137:** 384–90.

4. Bonadio WA. The cerebrospinal fluid: physiologic aspects and alterations associated with bacterial meningitis. *Pediatr Infect Dis J* 1992; **11:** 423–32.

5. Leist TP, Frei K, Kam-Hansen S, Zinkernagel RM, Fontana A. Tumor necrosis factor alpha in cerebrospinal fluid during bacterial, but not viral, meningitis. *J Exp Med* 1988; **167:** 1743–8.

6. McCracken GH, Mustafa MM, Ramilo O, Olsen KD, Risser RC. Cerebrospinal fluid interleukin 1-beta and tumor necrosis factor concentrations and outcome from neonatal gram-negative enteric bacillary meningitis. *Pediatr Infect Dis J* 1989; **8:** 155–9.

7. Nadal D, Leppert D, Frei K, Gallo P, Lamche H, Fontana A. Tumor necrosis factor alpha in infectious meningitis. *Arch Dis Child* 1989; **64:** 1274–9.

8. Mustafa MM, Lebel MH, Ramilo O, et al. Correlation of interleukin-1 beta and cachectin concentrations in cerebrospinal fluid and outcome from bacterial meningitis. *J Pediatr* 1989; **115:** 208–13.

9. Glimaker M, Kragsbjerg P, Forsgren M, Olcen P. Tumor necrosis factor-alpha (TNF alpha) in cerebrospinal fluid from patients with meningitis of different etiologies: high levels of TNF alpha indicate bacterial meningitis. *J Infect Dis* 1993; **167:** 882–9.

10. Johnson GM, McAbee GA, Seaton ED, Lipson SM. Suspect value of non-CSF viral cultures in the diagnosis of enteroviral CNS infection in young infants. *Dev Med Child Neurol* 1992; **34:** 876–84.

11. Ramilo O, Mustafa MM, Porter J, Saez-Llorens X, Mertsola J, Olsen KD, Luby JP, Beutler B, McCracken GH. Detection of interleukin 1-beta but not tumor necrosis factor-alpha in cerebrospinal fluid of children with aseptic meningitis. *Amer J Dis Child* 1990; **144:** 349–52.

12. Dussaix E, Lepon P, Ponsot G, Huault G, Tardieu M. Intrathecal synthesis of different alpha-interferons in patients with various neurologic diseases. *Acta Neurol Scand* 1985; **71:** 504–9.

13. Abbott RJ, Bolderson I, Gruer PJK. Assessment of an immunoassay for interferon-alpha in cerebrospinal fluid as a diagnostic aid in infections of the central nervous system. *J Infect* 1987; **15:** 153–60.

65.   *Arthropod-borne viruses that infect the CNS typically present as an acute viral encephalitis but may, in their milder forms, present as an aseptic meningitis*

Acute viral infections of the CNS are traditionally divided into two syndromes: meningitis and encephalitis, although meningoencephalitis is perhaps a better term as there is usually a meningeal reaction that accompanies the infectious process in the brain parenchyma. Arthropod-borne viruses (arboviruses) are transmitted to vertebrate hosts after an obligatory cycle in blood-sucking arthropods, including mosquitoes, ticks and sandflies.[1] The host is inoculated with infected saliva from the insect vector; the virus then replicates locally at the skin site. This is followed by a viremia with eventual spread of the virus to the CNS.[2] In the United States, the principal mosquito-borne viruses are the Eastern, Western and Venezuelan equine encephalitides (Alphaviruses), California encephalitis (a Bunyavirus) and St Louis encephalitis (a Flavivirus).[3] California and St Louis encephalitis are the most common and important causes of human arboviral encephalitis in the United States.[1] St Louis encephalitis occurs throughout the United States and Canada with epidemics typically in August through October. The infection may be asymptomatic or can present as fever, meningitis or encephalitis. This viral infection is often characterized by tremors involving the head and neck and upper extremities, and the syndrome of inappropriate secretion of antidiuretic hormone (SIADH).[1] Bunyaviridae infections may also present as an aseptic meningitis, especially the LaCrosse variety of the California Serogroup found in the Midwestern and Eastern United States. The LaCrosse virus was originally isolated from the brain of a patient from LaCrosse, Wisconsin.[4] Cases of California encephalitis occur between June and October and may present with seizures and focal neurologic signs resembling that of herpes simplex encephalitis.[1] The mortality rate from California encephalitis, however, is less than 1% and sequelae are rare.[5]

Eastern equine encephalitis is endemic along the coastal region of the Eastern and Gulf Coast of the United States, in the Caribbean and in Central and South America.[6] Eastern equine encephalitis is the most severe encephalitis caused by an arbovirus with a clinical presentation characterized by stupor and coma, generalized rigidity and seizures. The reported mortality rate is 50–75% with severe sequelae in survivors, especially in children, including mental retardation, seizures and paralysis.[1,7–9] Western equine encephalitis occurs in the western United States and Canada, Central America and northern South America. The infection may be asymptomatic, and neurologic manifestations are frequently very mild or absent, with seizures being most common in infants and young children. Upper respiratory tract or gastrointestinal symptoms predominate.[1] Venezuelan encephalitis occurs in Central and South America. Central nervous system infection typically presents as an aseptic meningitis with fever, myalgias and headache. Encephalitis occurs in a small percentage of patients.[10,11]

Central European encephalitis (CEE) virus is transmitted to man by a tick bite from the species *Ixodes ricinus*. An incubation period of 2–28 days is followed by nonspecific symptoms and signs, including fever, malaise, headache and fatigue. This initial stage lasts from 1 to 8 days and is followed by a fever-free and symptom-free interval of 1 to 20 days. Neurologic abnormalities may then develop, including meningitis, meningoencephalitis, meningomyelitis or meningoencephalomyelitis. The most frequent neurologic presentation of CEE in individuals younger than 40 years of age is meningitis. With increasing age, and especially in the elderly, severe clinical symptoms with paralysis may develop. The majority of individuals infected with the CEE virus have an asymptomatic infection with viremia only. Approximately one-third of infected persons develop neurologic abnormalities.[12]

Japanese encephalitis virus, a member of the St Louis complex of flaviviruses, is the most common cause of arthropod-borne human encephalitis worldwide.[13] Epidemic disease occurs throughout China, India and northern parts of Southeast Asia. In China alone, there are more than 10,000 cases annually, despite childhood immunization.[14] The major vectors of Japanese encephalitis virus are rice-field-breeding culicine mosquitoes. The virus reaches the brain by hematogenous dissemination and infects the basal ganglia, thalamus and nuclei of the brainstem. The involvement of the basal ganglia and thalamus explains the tremors seen during the acute disease, and the dystonic and parkinsonian sequelae seen in survivors.[13] A factor predictive of outcome is the rapid appearance of antibodies directed against Japanese B encephalitis in the CSF, which apparently lessen the severity of the disease.[14]

A general rule of thumb to distinguish clinically between viral meningitis and viral meningoencephalitis is that an altered level of consciousness, focal or multifocal neurologic signs, or seizures suggest a diagnosis of viral meningoencephalitis. The presence of headache, nuchal rigidity, photophobia and a normal level of consciousness is characteristic of viral meningitis. In both viral meningitis and viral meningoencephalitis, examination of the CSF demonstrates a mild-to-moderate pleocytosis with a predominance of lymphocytes or mononuclear cells, a mild elevation in the protein concentration and a normal glucose concentration. In cases of viral encephalitis, the electroencephalogram will show either focal or diffuse generalized slowing and may demonstrate focal spike or sharp wave discharges. The diagnosis is made by a four-fold or greater rise in the titer of viral antibodies between the acute and convalescent serology. The convalescent serology is typically obtained 4–6 weeks after an acute titer has been obtained. Viral cultures from throat, stool and the CSF should be obtained. Treatment is largely supportive.

References

1. Jackson AC, Johnson RT. Aseptic meningitis and acute viral encephalitis. In: McKendall RR (ed.), *Handbook of Clinical Neurology: Viral Disease*. Amsterdam: Elsevier, 1989; 125–48.
2. Johnson RT. Arboviral encephalitis. In: Warren KS, Mahmoud AAF (eds), *Tropical and Geographic Medicine*. New York: McGraw-Hill, 1990; 691–700.
3. Connolly KJ, Hammer SM. The acute aseptic meningitis syndrome. *Infect Dis Clin North Amer* 1990; **4:** 599–622.
4. Thompson WH, Kalfayan B, Anslow RO. Isolation of California encephalitis group virus from a fatal human illness. *Am J Epidemiol* 1965; **81:** 245–53.
5. Johnson KP, Lepow ML, Johnson RT. California encephalitis. I. Clinical and epidemiological studies. *Neurology* 1968; **18:** 250–4.
6. Shope RE. Alphaviruses. In: Fields BN (ed.), *Virology*. New York: Raven Press, 1985; 931–53.
7. Farber S, Hill A, Connerly ML, Dingle JH. Encephalitis in infants and children caused by the virus of the eastern variety of equine encephalitis. *JAMA* 1940; **114:** 1725–31.

8. Ayres JC, Feemster RF. The sequelae of eastern equine encephalomyelitis. *N Engl J Med* 1949; **240:** 960–2.
9. Feemster RF. Equine encephalitis in Massachusetts. *N Engl J Med* 1957; **257:** 701–4.
10. McConnell S, Spertzel RO. Venezuelan equine encephalomyelitis. In: Beran GW (ed.), *CRC Handbook Series in Zoonoses, Section B: Viral Zoonoses*, vol. 1. Boca Raton: CRC Press, 1981; 59–69.
11. Shope RE. Medical significance of togaviruses: an overview of diseases caused by togaviruses in man and in domestic and wild vertebrate animals. In: Schlesinger RW (ed.), *The Togaviruses, Biology, Structure, Replication*. New York: Academic Press, 1980; 47–82.
12. Tiecks F, Pfister HW, Ray CG. Other viral infections. In: Hacke W (ed.), *Neuro Critical Care*. Berlin: Springer-Verlag, 1994; 468–92.
13. Johnson RT. The pathogenesis of acute viral encephalitis and postinfectious encephalomyelitis. *J Infect Dis* 1987; **155:** 359–64.
14. Whitley RJ. Viral encephalitis. *N Engl J Med* 1990; **323:** 242–50.

66.   The combination of a facial nerve palsy and an aseptic meningitis is suggestive of Lyme disease

Lyme disease is a tick-transmitted multisystem disorder caused by the spirochete *Borrelia burgdorferi*. The characteristic skin lesion, erythema chronicum migrans (ECM), is often the first manifestation of Lyme disease. The skin lesion was initially recognized in Europe in 1910[1] and the associated neurologic abnormalities were first described in 1922.[2] Lyme disease was first recognized in the United States as the cause of epidemic arthritis in Lyme, Connecticut in 1975.[3]

Following introduction through the skin by the bite of an infected *Ixodes* tick, the organisms disseminate to many organs, including the central nervous system. There are several neurologic syndromes associated with Lyme disease, including:

1. headache with meningismus;
2. aseptic meningitis;
3. meningoencephalomyelitis;
4. cranial neuropathies;
5. radiculoneuritis;
6. muscle disorders;
7. a post-infectious syndrome characterized by persistent fatigue and difficulty with memory and concentration.[4]

The characteristic skin lesion, ECM, may be accompanied by secondary annular skin lesions, malaise and fatigue, headache, stiff neck, fever, myalgias, arthralgias, dysesthesias, sore throat, or abdominal pain.[5] During this early stage of Lyme disease, patients may complain of severe headache and stiff neck, but the CSF is typically normal.

Symptoms of Lyme meningitis begin a median of 4 weeks after the onset of ECM, and usually after a latent period, and are often accompanied by superimposed cranial and/or peripheral neuropathies. The predominant symptom is headache, which typically fluctuates in intensity. Additional symptoms of nausea and vomiting, photophobia, or pain on eye motion are not unusual. On physical examination, there is evidence of mild neck stiffness.[5] Facial nerve palsy, radicular symptoms and joint problems may also be seen at this stage.

Examination of the CSF demonstrates a mononuclear pleocytosis (generally less than 200 white blood cells/mm³), with occasional plasma cells and atypical lymphocytes. The protein concentration may be elevated, but is generally less than 100 mg/dL. A decreased CSF glucose concentration is unusual.[4] Intrathecal anti-*B. burgdorferi* antibodies are present in 70–90% of cases.[4,6,7] Cerebrospinal fluid protein concentrations are often higher in patients with radiculoneuritis than in those without it.[5] Patients may experience encephalitic symptoms – sleep disturbances, difficulty concentrating, poor memory, irritability, and emotional lability in addition to signs and symptoms of meningitis.[5] The electroencephalogram (EEG) may show slowing or poor regulation of the background activity. A more severe encephalitis is a rare complication of late infection.[4]

Radiculoneuritis is more common in Europe than in North America. In Europe, this illness has been given several different names including Bannwarth's syndrome, chronic meningitis and tick-borne meningopolyneuritis.[5,8] The syndrome consists of a painful peripheral neuropathy and a CSF lymphocytic pleocytosis. Cranial nerve involvement, most commonly facial palsy, occurs in approximately 40% of patients. Headache is unusual and neck stiffness is mild. Arthritis frequently accompanies Lyme disease in the United States, but is rarely present in the European form of this disease.[5]

The third generation cephalosporin, ceftriaxone, is the recommended antimicrobial agent for Lyme meningitis. The dose is 2 g/day for adults, and 75–100 mg/kg daily for children. Treatment is continued for at least 2 weeks.[4]

The following characteristics of the meningitis of Lyme disease are thought to be helpful in distinguishing meningitis due to *B. burgdorferi* from meningitis due to tuberculosis, fungal infections or sarcoidosis:

1. Lyme disease meningitis is generally not associated with significant meningismus, raised intracranial pressure, or hypoglycorrhachia.
2. Facial nerve palsy, including bilateral facial nerve palsy, is common in Lyme disease and, if present, often helps separate it from other entities.[5]

References

1. Afzelius A. Report to Verhandlungen der dermatologischen Gesellschaft zu Stockholm on December 16, 1909. *Arch Dermatol Syph* 1910; **101:** 405–6.
2. Garin-Bujadoux C. Paralysis par les tiques. *J Med Lyon* 1922; **71:** 765–7.
3. Steere AC, Malawista SE, Snydman DR, et al. Lyme arthritis: an epidemic of

oligoarticular arthritis in children and adults in three Connecticut communities. *Arthritis Rheum* 1977; **20:** 7–17.

4. Coyle PK. Neurologic Lyme disease. *Semin Neurol* 1992; **12:** 200–8.
5. Pachner AR, Steere AC. The triad of neurologic manifestations of Lyme disease: meningitis, cranial neuritis, and radiculoneuritis. *Neurology* 1985; **35:** 47–53.
6. Steere AC, Berardi VP, Weeks KE, et al. Evaluation of the intrathecal antibody response to *Borrelia burgdorferi* as a diagnostic test for Lyme neuroborreliosis. *J Infect Dis* 1990; **161:** 1203–9.
7. Halperin JJ, Volkman DJ, Wu P. Central nervous system abnormalities in Lyme neuroborreliosis. *Neurology* 1991; **41:** 1571–82.
8. Bannwarth A. Zur Klinic und Pathogenese der "chronischen lymphocytaren meningitis." *Arch Psychiatr Nervenkr* 1944; **117:** 161–85.

67. Meningeal involvement by sarcoidosis may present as an aseptic meningitis

Neurosarcoidosis is a disorder that affects 5% of all cases of sarcoidosis.[1-3] Meningeal involvement in sarcoidosis is a common pathologic finding. Cranial neuropathy is the most frequent manifestation of sarcoidosis of the nervous system, and a facial nerve palsy is the single most common abnormality.[2] Aseptic meningitis, characterized by headache, meningismus and a CSF lymphocytic pleocytosis, may be a recurrent problem in patients with neurosarcoidosis.[2] When a patient with systemic sarcoidosis develops an aseptic meningitis, the diagnosis of neurosarcoidosis is frequently considered. The more difficult clinical problem is ruling out neurosarcoidosis in the setting of an aseptic meningitis without established systemic sarcoidosis.

Sarcoidosis is defined as a multisystem granulomatous disorder of unknown etiology. It most commonly affects young adults, and presents with bilateral hilar lymphadenopathy, pulmonary infiltrates, skin or eye lesions. The diagnosis is established by histologic evidence of widespread noncaseating epithelioid-cell granulomas in more than one organ or a positive Kveim–Siltzbach skin-test.[2,4] A gallium scan is very useful to show multisystem involvement. The gallium scan may be positive, showing diffuse uptake in the lungs even in the absence of clinical involvement, and appears to be more sensitive than chest X-ray for sarcoidosis.[1,5,6] The combination of diffuse pulmonary uptake on gallium scanning and an elevated serum angiotensin converting enzyme has a high specificity (83–99%) for the diagnosis of sarcoidosis.[1,5] Biopsy of an enlarged lymph node, salivary gland, conjunctiva or skin lesion may provide histologic confirmation of sarcoidosis. A magnetic resonance scan is useful to demonstrate the extent of meningeal involvement as well as intracranial mass lesions, diencephalic disease and spinal cord lesions.

Patients with neurosarcoidosis may have an elevated IgG index and synthesis rate indicative of intrathecal immunoglobulin production.[7,8]

Oligoclonal banding has also been identified in the CSF of patients with neu-rosarcoidosis.[8,9] The CSF abnormalities in sarcoidosis are nonspecific, including an elevated protein concentration, a lymphocytic pleocytosis and a decreased glucose concentration. A measurement of the CSF angiotensin converting enzyme (ACE) may be helpful in making the diagnosis of neurosarcoidosis. Angiotensin converting enzyme is produced in the epithelioid and giant cells of sarcoid granulomas which are usually widespread throughout the meninges. Angiotensin converting enzyme has a molecular weight of 150,000 and, as it does not passively leak through the blood–brain barrier, its presence in CSF is due to synthesis in the CNS granulomas.[10] Several investigators have demonstrated significant elevations of CSF ACE activity in patients with neurosarcoidosis.[10-12] Normal CSF ACE values do not rule out neurosarcoidosis. Elevated CSF ACE values have been detected in patients with CNS infections and malignant tumors, though sarcoidosis was not considered in the differential diagnosis in these cases.[10] An elevation in the CSF ACE has also been reported in a few cases of multiple sclerosis, the Guillain–Barre syndrome and Behcet's disease.[11] The elevation of CSF ACE was generally greater in sarcoidosis than in other neurologic illnesses.[1,10,11]

Prednisone is generally recommended for initial therapy of neurosar-coidosis. The addition of immunosuppressive agents such as cyclosporin, azathioprine or cyclophosphamide may be efficacious in patients in whom steroid therapy fails or a reduction in the steroid dose is desirable.[1]

References

1. Scott TF. Neurosarcoidosis: Progress and clinical aspects. *Neurology* 1993; **43**: 8–12.
2. Stern BJ, Krumholz A, Johns C, Scott P, Nissim J. Sarcoidosis and its neurologic manifestations. *Arch Neurol* 1985; **42**: 909–17.
3. Delaney P. Neurologic manifestations of sarcoidosis: review of the literature, with a report of 23 cases. *Ann Intern Med* 1977; **87**: 336–46.
4. James DG, Turiaf J, Hosoda Y, et al. Description of sarcoidosis. Report of the subcommittee on classification and definition. *Ann NY Acad Sci* 1976; **278**: 742.
5. Nosal A, Schleissner LA, Mishkin FS, Lieberman J. Angiotensin-I-converting enzyme and gallium scan in noninvasive evaluation of sarcoidosis. *Ann Intern Med* 1979; **90**: 328–31.
6. Israel H, Gushue G, Park C. Assessment of gallium-67 scanning in pulmonary and extrapulmonary sarcoidosis. *Ann NY Acad Sci* 1986; **465**: 455–62.
7. Borucki SJ, Nguyen BV, Ladoulis CT, McKendall RR. Cerebrospinal fluid immunoglobulin abnormalities in neurosarcoidosis. *Arch Neurol* 1989; **46**: 270–3.
8. Scott TF, Seay AR, Goust JM. Pattern and concentration of IgG in cerebrospinal fluid in neurosarcoidosis. *Neurology* 1989; **39**: 1637–9.
9. Kinnman J, Link H. Intrathecal production of oligoclonal IgM and IgG in CNS sarcoidosis. *Acta Neurol Scand* 1984; **69**: 97–106.
10. Oksanen V, Fyhrquist F, Somer H, Gronhagen-Riska C. Angiotensin converting enzyme in cerebrospinal fluid: A new assay. *Neurology* 1985; **35**: 1220–3.
11. Schweisfurth H, Schioberg-Schiegnitz S, Kuhn W, Parusel B. Angiotensin-I-

converting enzyme in cerebrospinal fluid of patients with neurologic diseases. *Klin Wochenschr* 1987; **65**: 955–8.

12. Seem CPC, Norfolk G, Spokes EG. CSF angiotensin-converting enzyme in neurosarcoidosis. *Lancet* 1985; **i:** 456–7.

68.   *Migraine may be associated with a CSF lymphocytic pleocytosis, and aseptic meningitis may be associated with migraine-like attacks*

Over the last 20 years, a number of case reports have appeared in the literature of migraine-like headaches and CSF abnormalities. Examination of the CSF has demonstrated an elevated opening pressure, an elevated protein concentration and a lymphocytic pleocytosis.[1-4]

Under the new International Headache Society classification of headache, migraine is now subclassified as one of the following:

1. migraine without aura;
2. migraine with aura;
3. ophthalmoplegic migraine;
4. retinal migraine;
5. childhood periodic syndromes that may be precursors to or associated with migraine;
6. complications of migraine;
7. migrainous disorder.

Types of auras include the following:

1. homonymous visual disturbance;
2. unilateral paresthesias, numbness or both;
3. unilateral weakness;
4. aphasia or unclassifiable speech difficulties.

To be classified as a migraine headache without aura the following criteria must be met:

1. headache lasting 4 to 72 hours;
2. two of the following characteristics: unilateral location, pulsating quality, moderate or severe intensity (inhibits or prohibits daily activities) and aggravation by walking up and down stairs or similar routine physical activity;
3. at least one of the following: nausea and/or vomiting, or photophobia and phonophobia.

To characterize a headache as a migraine with aura the headache must have at least three of the following four characteristics:

1. one or more fully reversible aura symptoms indicating focal cerebral cortical and/or brainstem dysfunction;
2. at least one aura symptom developing gradually over more than 4 minutes or two or more symptoms occurring in succession;
3. no aura symptom lasting more than 60 minutes;
4. headache follows aura with a free interval of less than 60 minutes (it may also begin before or simultaneously with the aura).[5]

In the syndrome of migrainous symptoms with a lymphocytic CSF pleocytosis, the onset of the illness begins with either a focal neurologic deficit such as a hemisensory loss, hemiparesis, language or speech difficulty, or a visual disturbance, followed by headache. Some of the patients have fever early in the illness. Cerebrospinal fluid viral cultures are negative, and acute and convalescent serology for California virus, herpes simplex, mumps and St Louis and western equine encephalitides are negative. This syndrome is typically self-limiting, although the neurologic deficit and/or headache may recur in a series of attacks for a brief period of time.[3]

The argument has been made repeatedly that this syndrome is not a migraine with aura and CSF pleocytosis, but rather an aseptic meningitis with migraine-like symptomatology or Mollaret's meningitis. In 1944, Mollaret described a syndrome of recurrent benign endothelioleukocytic meningitis in three patients.[6] In 1961, Bruyn et al.[7] reviewed the published reports of Mollaret's meningitis, and in 1972 Hermans et al.[8] reviewed the essential features of this form of meningitis and added five cases of their own. Mollaret's meningitis consists of recurrent brief episodes of meningitis alternating with symptom-free intervals. The attacks occur suddenly, and the symptoms reach maximum intensity within a few hours. Signs and symptoms include headache, neck pain, backache, muscle aches and neck stiffness, which persist for 1–3 days; during the attacks, Kernig's and Brudzinski's signs are typically positive. Transitory neurologic abnormalities may occur. Fever (up to 104°F) is present during the episodes, and nausea and vomiting may occur. All these symptoms and signs disappear as rapidly as they develop, and the patient is symptom-free and entirely well until the next episode. There are no residual neurologic abnormalities. The abnormalities in the CSF are defined by "three stages of pleocytosis". During the first 12–24 hours, the CSF demonstrates a pleocytosis (up to several thousand cells/mm^3) with a predominance of polymorphonuclear neutrophils (PMNs) and a large type of cell which Mollaret called an "endothelial–leukocytic" cell. This is a mononuclear cell characterized by an irregular, vague outline of the nuclear and cytoplasmic membranes. These cells are difficult to identify because they rapidly disintegrate while being examined in the counting chamber. A number of these cells can be seen only as "ghosts" and they can rarely be detected after the first day of an attack. The PMNs disappear, and the pleocytosis becomes predominantly lymphocytic. The lymphocytic cells also rapidly disappear, and within a matter of days after an episode the pleocytosis has almost completely resolved.[8] This syndrome of migrainous symptoms and lymphocytic CSF pleocytosis has been called a benign syndrome; similarly, Mollaret's meningitis has been called a benign recurrent aseptic meningitis.[9] The syndrome of migrainous symptoms with a CSF lymphocytic pleocytosis is characterized by multiple migrainous attacks during a single, self-limited illness which lasts from 1 to 12 weeks. Patients with Mollaret's meningitis have recurrent, separate episodes of meningitis over a period of 1 year or more, with symptom-free intervals lasting weeks, months and sometimes years. They may also have prominent meningeal signs, which are not present in patients with a migrainous syndrome with CSF pleocytosis.[10]

It is recommended that patients who present with a combination of migrainous symptoms and a CSF lymphocytic pleocytosis have viral cultures and acute and convalescent serologic studies. Regardless of whether this is migraine with a CSF lymphocytic pleocytosis or is instead an aseptic meningitis with migrainous symptomatology, it is a self-limited illness and the prognosis is good.

References

1. Kremenitzer M, Golden GS. Hemiplegic migraine. Cerebrospinal fluid abnormalities. *J Pediatr* 1974; **85:** 139.
2. Schraeder PL, Burns RA. Hemiplegic migraine associated with an aseptic meningeal reaction. *Arch Neurol* 1980; **37:** 377–9.
3. Bartleson JD, Swanson JW, Whisnant JP. A migrainous syndrome with cerebrospinal fluid pleocytosis. *Neurology* 1981; **31:** 1257–62.
4. Lhermitte F, Marteau R, Roullet E. To the Editor. *Neurology* 1982; **32:** 1074.
5. Olesen J. Headache Classification Committee of the International Headache Society. Classification and diagnostic criteria for headache disorders, cranial neuralgia, and facial pain. *Cephalalgia*, 1988; **8**(suppl 7): 1–96.
6. Mollaret P. La meningite endothelio–leucocytaire multirecurrente benigne: syndrome nouveau ou maladie nouvelle? (Document cliniques.) *Rev Neurol* 1944; **76:** 57.
7. Bruyn G, Straathoff LJ, Raymakers GM. Mollaret's meningitis. Differential diagnosis and diagnostic pitfalls. *Neurology* 1962; **12:** 745–53.
8. Hermans PE, Goldstein NP, Wellman WE. Mollaret's meningitis and differential diagnosis of recurrent meningitis. *Am J Med* 1972; **52:** 128–39.
9. Galdi A. Benign recurrent aseptic meningitis. *Arch Neurol* 1979; **36:** 657–8.
10. Bartleson JD, Swanson JW, Whisnant JP. Reply from the authors. *Neurology* 1982; **32:** 1075.

69.   *The most common infectious etiology of eosinophilic meningitis is the helminthic parasite,* Angiostrongylus cantonensis

Angiostrongylus cantonensis has been called the principal etiologic agent of human eosinophilic meningitis. The first human case was detected in Taiwan in 1944.[1] Infection is usually acquired by accidental ingestion of infected larvae in terrestrial mollusks, vegetables contaminated by mollusk slime, infected flat worms, freshwater and terrestrial crabs, and freshwater shrimp. Eosinophilic meningitis due to *A. cantonensis* occurs principally in south-east Asia and throughout the Pacific Basin.[2] The African land snail (*Achatina fulica*) which is often consumed as a delicacy (escargots) can cause infection. Infected rats that are sequestered on commercial ships are the principal means of intercontinental migration of the parasite beyond the Indopacific area.[1] *Angiostrongylus cantonensis* has been found in infected rats in Madagascar, Cuba, Egypt, Puerto Rico, New Orleans, Louisiana, Reunion Island and Côte d'Ivoire.[1]

The three major parasites that cause eosinophilic meningitis are *A. cantonensis*, *Baylisascaris procyonis* and *Gnathostoma spinigerum*. Meningitis results from the migration of larvae into the brain, which is often the consequence of migration into neuro-ocular tissue and/or along a nerve. *Baylisascaris procyonis* is a parasite of raccoons; people become infected from raccoon feces. Infection with *Gnathostoma spinigerum* is usually acquired from raw fish dishes such as somfak and sashimi. Infection with *A. cantonensis* most typically presents as a transient meningitis or, less commonly, as a more severe disease involving the brain, spinal cord and nerve roots. The most common presenting symptom is severe headache.[3] Meningismus, nausea and vomiting, and paresthesias are also common.[2] The characteristic presentation of CNS infection with *G. spinigerum* is the sudden onset of severe radicular pain or headache which may be followed by paralysis of the extremities or cranial nerves. An eosinophilic meningoencephalitis is typical of infection with *G. spinigerum* and is a much more fulminant illness than the meningitis due to *A. cantonensis*.[2,4] Eosinophilic meningitis due to *B. procyonis* is rare in humans, however it is expected that the incidence of this infection will increase in the United States due to the prevalence of infection in raccoons and their proximity to humans in many rural and suburban areas. In the two reported cases in humans, this infection presented as a meningoencephalitis and was fatal.[2,5,6]

Examination of the CSF in *A. cantonensis* meningitis demonstrates a mild-to-moderate pleocytosis with an eosinophilia exceeding 10% in 95% of cases, and typically in the range of 20–70%. Peripheral blood eosinophilia usually accompanies the eosinophilic pleocytosis in CSF. *Angiostrongylus cantonensis* has rarely been recovered from CSF. Several serologic tests have been developed, but have yet to be extensively evaluated. In most cases this is a self-limited disease and patients recover completely. Therapy with antihelminthic agents has no proven efficacy. Corticosteroids may be efficacious in severe infections.[2] The diagnosis of *G. spinigerum* meningitis is based on the abrupt onset of symptoms, the prominence of nerve root pain, evidence of eosinophilia in blood and CSF and, in some cases, areas of hemorrhage on computed tomography scans.[2] Therapy with a course of corticosteroids is recommended. The diagnosis of *B. procyonis* eosinophilic meningoencephalitis is made by the clinical presentation, a blood and CSF eosinophilia and a possible exposure to raccoon-contaminated soil. Therapy with a benzimidazole antihelminthic agent and a course of corticosteroids is recommended.[2]

There are other etiologies of eosinophilic meningitis in addition to infection with helminthic parasites. A CSF eosinophilia has been reported in as many as 35% of cases of neurocysticercosis.[7,8] A CSF eosinophilia has been reported in CNS coccidioidomycosis and cryptococcosis, although this is uncommon.[9,10] The infectious and less common noninfectious etiologies of eosinophilic meningitis are listed in Table 69.1.

Table 69.1   Eosinophilic meningitis

Infectious etiologies
Angiostrongylus cantonensis
Gnathostoma spinigerum
Baylisascaris procyonis
Cysticercosis
Cryptococcus neoformans
Coccidioides immites

Noninfectious etiologies
Idiopathic hypereosinophilic syndrome
Ventriculoperitoneal shunt
Hodgkin's disease
Nonsteroidal anti-inflammatory agents (ibuprofen)
Antimicrobial agents: parenteral ciprofloxacin,
    intraventricular vancomycin or gentamicin
Myelography with contrast agent
Sarcoidosis

Adapted from Weller and Liu (1993).[2]

References

1. Kliks MM, Palumbo NE. Eosinophilic meningitis beyond the Pacific Basin: the global dispersal of a peridomestic zoonosis caused by *Angiostrongylus cantonensis*, the nematode lungworm of rats. *Soc Sci Med* 1992; **34:** 199–212.
2. Weller PF, Liu LX. Eosinophilic meningitis. *Sem Neurol* 1993; **13:** 161–8.
3. Kuberski T, Wallace GD. Clinical manifestations of eosinophilic meningitis due to *Angiostrongylus cantonensis. Neurology* 1979; **29:** 1566–70.

4. Punyagupta S, Bunnag T, Juttijudata P. Eosinophilic meningitis in Thailand. Clinical and epidemiologic characteristics of 162 patients with myeloencephalitis probably caused by *Gnathostoma spinigerum*. *J Neurol Sci* 1990; **96:** 241–56.
5. Fox AS, Kazacos KR, Gould NS, et al. Fatal eosinophilic meningoencephalitis and visceral larval migrans caused by the raccoon ascarid *Baylisascaris procyonis*. *N Engl J Med* 1985; **312:** 1619–23.
6. Huff DS, Neafie RC, Binder MJ, et al. Case 4. The first fatal *Baylisascaris* infection in humans: an infant with eosinophilic meningoencephalitis. *Pediatr Pathol* 1984; **2:** 345–52.
7. Loo L, Braude A. Cerebral cysticercosis in San Diego. A report of 23 cases and a review of the literature. *Medicine* 1982; **61:** 341–59.
8. Torrealba G, Del Villar S, Tagle P, et al. Cysticercosis of the central nervous system: clinical and therapeutic considerations. *J Neurol Neurosurg Psychiatr* 1984; **47:** 784–90.
9. Muller W, Schorre W, Suchenwirth R, et al. A case of fatal cryptococcus meningitis with intraventricular granuloma. *Acta Neurochir* (Wien) 1978; **44:** 223–35.
10. Schermoly MJ, Hinthorn DR. Eosinophilia in coccidioidomycosis. *Arch Intern Med* 1988; **148:** 895–6.

9
Fungal Meningitis

70. *Suspect a fungal infection in neutropenic patients with persistent fever*

Fungal meningitis occurs primarily, but not solely, in individuals who are in a state of immunosuppression due to one of the following:

1. the acquired immune deficiency syndrome (AIDS);
2. organ transplantation;
3. immunosuppressive chemotherapy or chronic corticosteroid therapy;
4. lymphoreticular malignancies.

The most common fungi causing meningitis are *Cryptococcus neoformans* and *Coccidioides immites*, although other pathogens such as *Histoplasma capsulatum*, *Blastomyces dermatitidis*, *Sporothrix schenckii* and *Candida* species are increasingly reported. The incidence of cryptococcal meningitis has increased greatly due to the frequency of this infection in individuals with AIDS. The type of fungus causing the CNS infection can be predicted based on the type of underlying immune deficiency. Individuals with defects in cell-mediated immunity are at risk of infection with *C. neoformans*, *C. immites* and *H. capsulatum*. Individuals with granulocytopenia are at risk of infections due to *Candida* and *Aspergillus fumigatus*, and the *Zygomycetes* organisms (mucormycosis).[1]

Cryptococcus neoformans is a yeast-like fungus found in pigeon droppings, decaying fruit and vegetables, milk and soil. Systemic disease develops following inhalation of unencapsulated yeast. Human-to-human transmission does not occur. For unknown reasons, *C. neoformans* has a predilection for the CNS and spreads from a primary pulmonary infection to the meninges by hematogenous dissemination. The fungus develops a polysaccharide capsule in infected tissues. This allows for the antigenic identification of the organism in CSF.[2] Cryptococcal meningitis may occur as the AIDS-defining illness.[3] Cryptococcal meningitis, however, is rare in children with AIDS.[4] *Cryptococcus neoformans* is the most common cause of CNS infection in the transplant patient.[5]

Coccidioides immites is a dimorphic fungus that grows as a mold in the environment and as a yeast-like structure in human tissue. It is endemic to the desert areas of the south-west United States, specifically California, Arizona, New Mexico and Texas. The disease is acquired by inhaling the infectious particles. The initial pulmonary infection may be asymptomatic or may manifest with flu-like symptoms. Less than 1% of individuals who develop a primary infection will develop disseminated disease. Infection spreads to the meninges by hematogenous dissemination, which usually occurs within 3–6 months after the initial infection.[2] Associated conditions that increase the risk for meningitis include the following:

1. pregnancy;
2. hemodialysis;
3. immunosuppressive chemotherapy (in particular, corticosteroids);
4. organ transplantation;
5. AIDS.[6]

Infection with *Histoplasma capsulatum* is typically a benign self-limited and often asymptomatic disease. Many individuals in an endemic area will have a positive skin test to histoplasmin.[2] Disseminated disease occurs principally in individuals with impaired cell-mediated immunity. Immunosuppression is a risk factor for meningitis.[7] *Histoplasma capsulatum* is endemic to the Midwestern United States, principally the Mississippi, Ohio and St Lawrence river basins and in the Appalachian Mountains. The fungus is found in the soil, and avian and bat excrement help accelerate mycelial growth and spore formation. The spores become aerosolized and are inhaled. Like coccidioidomycosis, the initial pulmonary infection is generally benign. Hematogenous dissemination to the CNS is primarily to the meninges at the base of the brain.[2]

 Candida species may also cause CNS infection in the immunocompromised patient and this typically takes the form of a subacute or chronic meningitis. Meningitis typically develops in the setting of disseminated candidal infection during which the meninges become seeded during fungemia. Fungemia with meningitis due to this organism occurs most frequently under the following conditions:

1. central line infections, particularly those used for central hyperalimentation;
2. surgical manipulation of a colonized genitourinary tract or gastrointestinal tract;
3. hematogenous dissemination from a gastrointestinal site;
4. broad-spectrum antimicrobial therapy;
5. corticosteroid therapy.[5]

References

1. Pruitt AA. Central nervous system infections in cancer patients. *Neurol Clin* 1991; **9**: 867–88.
2. Treseler CB, Sugar AM. Fungal meningitis. *Infect Dis Clin North Amer* 1990; **4**: 789–808.
3. Shaunak S, Cohen J. Clinical management of fungal infection in patients with AIDS. *J Antimicrob Chemo* 1991; **28**(suppl A): 67–81.
4. Pizzo PA, Eddy J, Faloon J. Acquired immune deficiency syndrome in children:

Current problems and therapeutic considerations. *Am J Med* 1988; **85:** 195–202.

5. Conti DJ, Rubin RH. Infection of the central nervous system in organ transplant recipients. *Neurol Clin* 1988; **6:** 241–60.

6. Ampel NM, Wieden MA, Galgiani JN. Coccidioidomycosis: clinical update. *Rev Infect Dis* 1989; **6:** 897–911.

7. Wheat JJ, Batteiger BE, Sathapatayavongs B. *Histoplasma capsulatum* infections of the central nervous system: a clinical review. *Medicine* 1990; **69:** 244–60.

71.   *Headache and fever are the most common symptoms of fungal meningitis*

Cryptococcal meningitis may present as an acute illness with fever, headache, photophobia and an altered sensorium, or as an indolent illness with headache and low-grade fever. Because the fungi have a tendency to infect the basilar meninges, fungal meningitis may also present with cranial nerve palsies. There may be a history of a preceding pulmonary infection or skin lesion.[1,2] The clinical presentation of fungal meningitis in the organ transplant recipient may be extremely subtle due to the patient's impaired inflammatory response secondary to immunosuppressive therapy. The duration of immunosuppressive therapy is directly related to the risk of developing meningitis. Six months or more of immunosuppressive therapy is typically required in renal transplant patients before *Cryptococcus neoformans* meningitis develops. Chronic headache and fever are often the only clinical manifestations of the presence of meningitis in these patients. Cryptococcal skin lesions may precede the development of meningitis. They have an appearance ranging from papular or nodular lesions to a frank cellulitis (Fig. 71.1). The identification of cryptococcal skin lesions is an indication for lumbar puncture even in the absence of signs and symptoms of meningitis.[3]

Like CNS cryptococcal infection, CNS coccidioidomycosis may present as an acute illness or follow a subacute chronic course. The most common presenting symptoms are headache, low-grade fever, nausea and vomiting, and mental status changes. In the presence of a focal space occupying lesion or vasculitis, focal neurologic deficits and seizures may be part of the presenting symptomatology. Signs of meningeal irritation such as nuchal rigidity are usually absent.[4]

Meningitis is the predominant clinical manifestation of CNS histoplasmosis. Mental status abnormalities are common, including stupor, confusion, personality changes and cognitive deficits. Fever is present in nearly all cases. Headache is a very common symptom but meningismus is rare. Cranial nerve deficits involving the third, sixth and seventh cranial nerves may occur.[5]

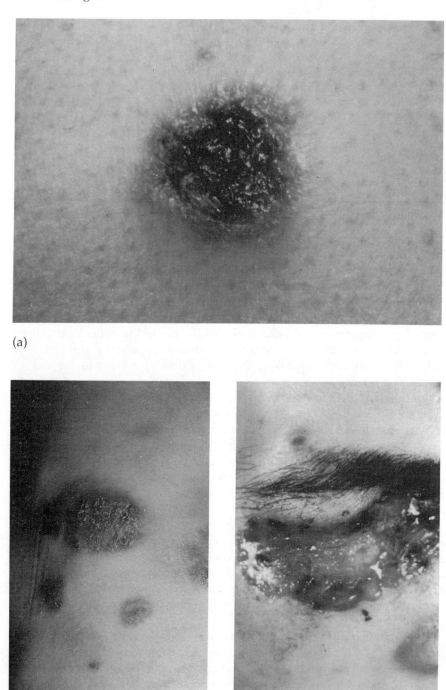

(a)

(b)   (c)

Fig. 71.1   (a, b and c) Cryptococcal skin lesions.

References

1. Shaunak S, Cohen J. Clinical management of fungal infection in patients with AIDS. *J Antimicrob Chemo* 1991; **28**(suppl A): 67–81.
2. Clark RA, Greer D, Atkinson W, Valainis GT, Hyslop N. Spectrum of *Cryptococcus neoformans* infection in 68 patients infected with human immunodeficiency virus. *Rev Infect Dis* 1990; **12**: 768–77.
3. Conti DJ, Rubin RH. Infection of the central nervous system in organ transplant recipients. *Neurol Clin* 1988; **6**: 241–60.
4. Treseler CB, Sugar AM. Fungal meningitis. *Infect Dis Clin North Amer* 1990; **4**: 789–808.
5. Wheat JJ, Batteiger BE, Sathapatayavongs B. *Histoplasma capsulatum* infections of the central nervous system: a clinical review. *Medicine* 1990; **69**: 244–60.

72.   *Fungi are difficult to isolate from CSF*

When fungal meningitis is suspected, CSF examination must be performed. However, caution must be exercised in performing a lumbar puncture in this patient population. Because fungal meningitis is so commonly associated with a state of immunosuppression, with neutropenia and thrombocytopenia, a platelet count should be obtained prior to lumbar puncture. Platelet transfusion should be performed before lumbar puncture for a platelet count of 50,000/mm^3 or less.[1] A neuroimaging procedure is recommended before lumbar puncture is performed in patients suspected of having fungal meningitis because of the high incidence of intracerebral mass lesions with CNS histoplasmosis and coccidioidomycosis. A neuroimaging study, either a cranial computed tomography (CT) scan or magnetic resonance imaging (MRI); is particularly important prior to lumbar puncture in patients with acquired immune deficiency syndrome (AIDS) because of the occurrence of CNS toxoplasmosis in these patients without focal neurologic deficits.[2] The kind of urgency for diagnosis and treatment of bacterial meningitis is not the same in cases of suspected fungal meningitis. Untreated fungal meningitis is not associated with the kind of rapid mortality that occurs in untreated bacterial meningitis. Bacterial meningitis is uncommon in human immunodeficiency virus-positive (HIV-positive) patients, therefore, either a CT scan or MRI is recommended before lumbar puncture is performed in this patient population.[2]

The CSF abnormalities in cryptococcal meningitis are the following:

1. a normal or slightly elevated opening pressure;
2. a lymphocytic pleocytosis;
3. an elevated protein concentration;
4. a decreased glucose concentration.

The CSF chemistry and cell counts may be normal in HIV-positive patients.

An India ink stain is reported to be positive in 50% of HIV-negative individuals, but positive in 75–88% of HIV-positive individuals.[2-4] Latex agglutination testing for the cryptococcal antigen is highly sensitive and specific and should be performed on all CSF specimens. *Cryptococcus neoformans* should grow in culture in 3–10 days.[3] Serum cryptococcal antigen titers are also often positive in patients with cryptococcal meningitis. However, the serum antigen titer is an indicator of systemic cryptococcal infection and has not been found to have predictive value for the subsequent development of *C. neoformans* meningitis. The serum antigen titers are useful in helping to monitor the response to induction therapy and for monitoring the response to low-dose maintenance therapy in suppressing disease, but should be used in conjunction with the clinical evaluation of the patient and CSF culture results.[2,5]

The CSF abnormalities in *Coccidioides immitis* meningitis are:

1. an elevated opening pressure;
2. a lymphocytic pleocytosis;
3. an elevated protein concentration;
4. decreased glucose concentration.

The organism grows rapidly and visible cultures can often be seen within 3 days, though large volumes of CSF are often necessary to isolate the organism.[3,6] The complement fixation antibody in the CSF is reported to have a specificity of 100% but a sensitivity of 75% in the setting of active disease.[3]

The characteristic CSF abnormalities in *Histoplasna capsulatum* meningitis are:

1. a CSF lymphocytic pleocytosis with cell counts less than 100/mm³, either neutrophils or lymphocytes predominate;
2. an elevated protein concentration;
3. a decreased glucose concentration.[7]

Culture of CSF is positive in 25–50% of cases, typically requiring as long as 45 days to grow. *Histoplasma capsulatum* is rarely seen on CSF smears.

It is recommended that large volumes of CSF be cultured on at least three occasions to increase the yield for isolation of fungi. In cases where multiple cultures of CSF obtained from a lumbar puncture are negative and the clinical findings suggest the possibility of fungal meningitis, CSF should be obtained by a cisternal puncture before empiric antifungal treatment is initiated or meningeal biopsy is performed. Meningeal biopsy for fungal meningitis is rarely positive for two reasons:

1. The basilar meninges are the typical area of infection by the fungus and a biopsy of the basilar meninges is difficult to perform and carries a high morbidity.
2. Although biopsy of the meninges overlying the cerebral hemispheres is more readily accessible than biopsy of the basilar meninges, the meninges overlying the cerebral hemispheres are typically normal in fungal meningitis.

Serologic tests for anti-*H. capsulatum* antibodies may be useful but should be interpreted with caution. This test has been reported to be negative in 10–25% of patients with disseminated histoplasmosis and falsely positive in patients with tuberculosis and other fungal infections due to cross reactivity between the anti-*H. capsulatum* antibodies and antigens from other organisms. Anti-*H. capsulatum* antibodies remain elevated for years following recovery from histoplasmosis and therefore may lead to an erroneous diagnosis of the present neurologic illness if not interpreted cautiously.

Histoplasma polysaccharide antigen (HPA) can be measured in urine, blood and CSF. This test has the same diagnostic significance as detection of the cryptococcal polysaccharide antigen in patients with cryptococcal meningitis. This test, however, is not widely available and it may be necessary to send specimens for HPA assay to a special laboratory.[7] Laboratory tests that may be helpful in addition to CSF analysis in making a diagnosis of fungal meningitis are listed in Table 72.1.

Table 72.1   Ancillary diagnostic tests for central nervous system fungal infections

Fungus	Diagnostic test
Cryptococcus neoformans	Serum cryptococcal antigen Culture blood, urine, sputum, bone marrow Biopsy skin lesions
Coccidiodes immites	Serum eosinophilia Chest X-ray
Histoplasma capsulatum	*Histoplasma* polysaccharide antigen (HPA) – urine, blood Chest X-ray Blood, urine and sputum cultures
Candida	Biopsy skin lesions Culture catheters
Aspergillus	Blood culture Chest X-ray Computed tomography of paranasal sinuses Biopsy skin lesions
Phycomycetes (Mucormycetes)	Computed tomography of paranasal sinuses Biopsy of black eschar

References

1. Pruitt AA. Central nervous system infection in cancer patients. *Neurol Clin* 1991; **9:** 867–88.
2. Shaunak S, Cohen J. Clinical management of fungal infection in patients with

AIDS. *J Antimicrob Chemo* 1991; **28**(suppl A): 67–81.
3. Treseler CB, Sugar AM. Fungal meningitis. *Infect Dis Clin North Amer* 1990; **4:** 789–808.
4. Chuck SL, Sande MA. Infection with *Cryptococcus neoformans* in the acquired immunodeficiency syndrome. *N Engl J Med* 1989; **321:** 794–9.
5. Nelson MR, Bower M, Smith D, Reed C, Shanson D, Gazzard B. The value of serum cryptococcal antigen in the diagnosis of cryptococcal infection in patients infected with the human immunodeficiency virus. *J Infect* 1990; **21:** 175–81.
6. Ampel NM, Wieden MA, Galgiani JN. Coccidioidomycosis: clinical update. *Rev Infect Dis* 1989; **6:** 897–911.
7. Wheat JJ, Batteiger BE, Sathapatayavongs B. *Histoplasma capsulatum* infections of the central nervous system: a clinical review. *Medicine* 1990; **69:** 244–60.

73.   Cryptococcus neoformans *is the most frequent causative agent of fungal meningitis in HIV-infected individuals*

Cryptococcus neoformans ranks third in frequency behind the human immunodeficiency virus (HIV) and *Toxoplasma gondii* in causing CNS infections in patients with acquired immune deficiency syndrome (AIDS).[1] Meningitis is the most common CNS infection caused by this fungus. The clinical presentation of cryptococcal meningitis in this patient population may be subtle. The most common symptoms are fatigue, headache, fever and cranial nerve deficits.[2] Fever and headache are present in 80–90% of patients.[1]

Meningitis due to *Coccidioides immitis* or *Histoplasma capsulatum* should be considered in HIV-positive individuals who live in areas endemic for these fungi. The endemic area for *C. immitis* is the south-west United States, and the endemic area for *H. capsulatum* is the Midwest United States and the Appalachian Mountain Region.[3]

References

1. Dismukes WE. Cryptococcal meningitis in patients with AIDS. *J Infect Dis* 1988; **157:** 624–8.
2. Chuck SL, Sande MA. Infections with *Cryptococcus neoformans* in the acquired immunodeficiency syndrome. *N Engl J Med* 1989; **321:** 794–9.
3. Clifford DB, Campbell JW. Management of neurologic opportunistic disorders in human immunodeficiency virus infection. *Semin Neurol* 1992; **12:** 28–33.

74.   *The CSF cryptococcal antigen is the best diagnostic test for cryptococcal meningitis*

The characteristic CSF abnormalities of fungal meningitis – lymphocytic pleocytosis, elevated protein and decreased glucose concentration – are not reliably present in cryptococcal meningitis in individuals who are infected with the human immunodeficiency virus (HIV).[1] The CSF cryptococcal antigen assay is highly sensitive and can be detected in CSF in 95% of cases of cryptococcal meningitis in patients with acquired immune deficiency syndrome (AIDS), and 85–90% of cases of cryptococcal meningitis overall.[2] *Cryptococcus neoformans* can also be identified on India ink stain, but large volumes (40–50 mL) of CSF are often required to identify the organism and grow it in culture. Consideration should be given to obtaining CSF by cisternal or high cervical puncture if a fungal infection is highly probable and the organism has not been recovered from CSF obtained by lumbar puncture.[2]

The CSF cryptococcal antigen titer can be used to follow therapy in non-AIDS patients. Following a recommended course of therapy, a negative CSF cryptococcal antigen titer or a low titer suggests the infection has been successfully treated. In AIDS patients, the initial CSF cryptococcal antigen titer and subsequent titers obtained during and following treatment have not been found to have prognostic significance.[3,4] The CSF cryptococcal antigen test may remain positive in AIDS patients despite adequate treatment and may represent the release of free antigen from dead cells or the slow clearance of the polysaccharide antigen from the CSF rather than an ongoing fungal infection.[5]

Serum cryptococcal antigen titers may be useful in monitoring the efficacy of low-dose therapy in suppressing disease. High or increasing titers during maintenance therapy should be considered evidence of failure or relapse only when they have been confirmed by a change in the patient's clinical status or by the presence of positive cultures.[5]

References

1. Clifford DB, Campbell JW. Management of neurologic opportunistic disorders in human immunodeficiency virus infection. *Semin Neurol* 1992; **12**: 28–33.
2. Greenlee JE. Approach to diagnosis of meningitis: cerebrospinal fluid evaluation. *Infect Dis Clin North Amer* 1990; **4**: 583–98.
3. Treseler CB, Sugar AM. Fungal meningitis. *Infect Dis Clin North Amer* 1990; **4**: 789–808.
4. Chuck SL, Sande MA. Infection with *Cryptococcus neoformans* in the acquired immunodeficiency syndrome. *N Engl J Med* 1989; **321**: 794–9.
5. Shaunak S, Cohen J. Clinical management of fungal infection in patients with AIDS. *J Antimicrob Chemo* 1991; **28**(suppl A): 67–81.

75.   *Intravenous amphotericin B has been the gold standard for the treatment of fungal meningitis*

Cryptococcal meningitis in immunocompetent patients is treated with either intravenous amphotericin B (0.4–0.6 mg/kg/day) for 10 weeks, or intravenous amphotericin B (0.3 mg/kg/day) *and* oral flucytosine (150 mg/kg/day) for 6 weeks (Table 75.1).[1-3] A test dose of 1 mg of amphotericin B is administered initially. Therapy is initiated with a dose of 0.25 mg/kg with slow daily titrations to the target dose.

Table 75.1   Recommended therapy of fungal meningitis

Organism	Antifungal agent
Cryptococcus neoformans Non-AIDS patient	Intravenous amphotericin B 0.3 mg/kg/day *plus* Flucytosine 150 mg/kg/day for 6 weeks *or* Intravenous amphotericin B 0.4–0.6 mg/kg/day
AIDS patient	Intravenous amphotericin B (0.5–0.8 mg/kg/day) for a total dose of 1–1.5 g followed by chronic suppressive therapy with fluconazole (200 mg/day)
Cocccidioides immites	Intravenous amphotericin B 0.4–0.6 mg/kg/day *plus* Intraventricular amphotericin B 0.25–0.75 mg three times weekly
Histoplasma capsulatum	Intravenous amphotericin B for a total dose of 35 mg/kg administered over 6–12 weeks

The main adverse effect of amphotericin B is nephrotoxicity, which develops in 80% of patients. Renal function should be monitored two or three times a week during the first month and then weekly for the duration of therapy. This should include urinalysis, serum creatinine, blood urea nitrogen, serum potassium, sodium and magnesium, bicarbonate and hematocrit.[4] Fever, shaking chills and hypotension may occur during the infusion of this drug. The addition of flucytosine allows for a reduction in the dose of amphotericin B and, therefore, potentially a decrease in the nephrotoxicity of this drug. Major toxic effects of flucytosine are bone marrow suppression (anemia, leukopenia, thrombocytopenia) and hepatitis. The adverse effects of flucytosine occur when serum concentrations of the drug exceed 100 µg/mL; therefore, serum concentrations of this drug need to be monitored on a regular basis.[4,5]

The oral antifungal agent, ketoconazole, is not recommended for the therapy of cryptococcal meningitis because this agent does not readily cross the blood–brain barrier and high doses are poorly tolerated.[6]

Cryptococcal meningitis in patients with acquired immune deficiency syndrome (AIDS) is treated for at least 6 weeks with intravenous amphotericin B for a total dose of at least 1–1.5 g, followed by chronic suppressive therapy with fluconazole at a dosage of 200 mg/day (Table 75.1).[3,7,8] The addition of flucytosine to amphotericin B did not enhance survival in one retrospective study.[9] The bone marrow toxicity of flucytosine is a major problem in AIDS patients who are already receiving other antiviral agents that also cause bone marrow suppression. Orally administered fluconazole can be used as primary therapy of cryptococcal meningitis in patients with AIDS, but is only presently recommended for patients who are at low risk for treatment failure. Patients at low risk for treatment failure have a normal mental status pretreatment, a CSF cryptococcal antigen titer below 1:1024 and a CSF white blood cell count above $0.02 \times 10^9/L$.[10]

Patients with AIDS who have been treated successfully for cryptococcal meningitis most frequently relapse due to clinically silent persistent or recurrent urinary cryptococcosis. Cultures of urine obtained after prostatic massage should be part of the assessment of patients who have completed their induction therapy.[7,11]

References

1. Gallis HA, Drew RH, Pickard WW. Amphotericin B: 30 years of clinical experience. *Rev Infect Dis* 1990; **12**: 308–29.
2. Bennett JE, Dismukes WE, Duma RJ, Medoff G, et al. A comparison of amphotericin B alone and combined with flucytosine in the treatment of cryptococcal meningitis. *N Engl J Med* 1979; **301**: 126–31.
3 Dismukes WE, Cloud G, Gallis HA, et al. Treatment of cryptococcal meningitis with combination amphotericin B and flucytosine for four as compared with six weeks. *N Engl J Med* 1987; **317**: 334–41.
4. Sugar AM, Stern JJ, Dupont B. Overview: treatment of cryptococcal meningitis. *Rev Infect Dis* 1990; **12**: 5338–48.
5. Kauffman CA, Frame PT. Bone marrow toxicity associated with 5-fluorocytosine therapy. *Antimicrob Agents Chemother* 1977; **11**: 244–7.
6. Sugar AM, Alsip SG, Galgiani JN, Graybill JR, Dismukes WE, Cloud GA, Craven PC, Stevens DA. Pharmacology and toxicity of high-dose ketoconazole. *Antimicrob Agents Chemother* 1987; **31**: 1874–8.
7. Bozzette SA, Larsen RA, Chiu J, Leal MAE, et al. A placebo-controlled trial of maintenance therapy with fluconazole after treatment of cryptococcal meningitis in the acquired immunodeficiency syndrome. *N Engl J Med* 1991; **324**: 580–4.
8. Powderly WG, Saag MS, Cloud GA, Robinson P. A controlled trial of fluconazole

or amphotericin B to prevent relapse of cryptococcal meningitis in patients with the acquired immunodeficiency syndrome. *N Engl J Med* 1992; **326:** 793–8.

9. Chuck SL, Sande MA. Infections with *Cryptococcus neoformans* in the acquired immunodeficiency syndrome. *N Engl J Med* 1989; **321:** 794–9.

10. Saag MS, Powderly WG, Cloud GA, Robinson P. Comparison of Amphotericin B with fluconazole in the treatment of acute AIDS-associated cryptococcal meningitis. *N Engl J Med* 1992; **326:** 83–9 .

11. Shaunak S, Cohen J. Clinical management of fungal infection in patients with AIDS. *J Antimicrob Chemo* 1991; **28**(suppl A): 67–81.

76.　*Repeat examination of the CSF is not necessary to monitor response to treatment of cryptococcal meningitis*

The clinical status of the patient is the best indicator of response to therapy. A repeat examination of the CSF is not indicated if the patient has improved clinically.

The serum cryptococcal antigen titer can be expected to decrease by at least four dilutions after successful therapy of this infection.[1]

The CSF should be re-examined if there is a recurrence of symptoms. The cryptococcal antigen titer can remain positive despite successful treatment, but positive fungal cultures imply treatment failure or relapse.[1]

References

1. McArthur JC. Neurologic diseases associated with human immunodeficiency virus type 1 infection. In: Johnson RT, Griffin JW (eds), *Current Therapy in Neurologic Disease*. St Louis, MO: *Mosby Year Book*, 1993; 146–52.

77.　*Coccidioides meningitis must be treated with intrathecal and intravenous amphotericin B*

Patients infected with the human immunodeficiency virus (HIV) and organ transplant recipients are at increased risk for severe disseminated coccidioidomycosis with involvement of the CNS. Most cases in both patient populations are thought to be due to reactivation of infection rather than to newly acquired infection.[1,2] Intrathecal plus intravenous amphotericin B is the only established treatment of coccidioidal meningitis.[1] Amphotericin B is administered either through an Ommaya reservoir or by intracisternal injection at a dosage of 0.25–0.75 mg 3 times weekly for 3 months followed by a tapering course. Therapy is started at a dose of 0.1 mg/day, and the dose is slowly titrated, as tolerated, up to a dosage of 0.5–0.75 mg every other day.

It is recommended that treatment be continued for at least a year after obtaining a normal CSF, and that the CSF be examined at 6-week intervals for 2 years after the end of treatment.[3,4] The addition of intrathecal hydrocortisone or methylprednisolone to intrathecal amphotericin B may reduce drug-related inflammation.[1,5] Fluconazole therapy, 400–800 mg daily for 12 months or longer, has been successful in treating some cases of coccidioidal meningitis.[6] Fluconazole can also be used for continual suppressive therapy for life for coccidioidomycoses in individuals infected with human immunodeficiency virus.[7]

References

1. Ampel NM, Wieden MA, Galgiani JN. Coccidioidomycosis: clinical update. *Rev Infect Dis* 1989; **11:** 897–911.
2. Shaunak S, Cohen J. Clinical management of fungal infection in patients with AIDS. *J Antimicrob Chemo* 1991; **28**(suppl A): 67–81.
3. Perfect JR. Diagnosis and treatment of fungal meningitis. In: Scheld WM, Whitley RJ, Durack DT (eds) *Infections of the Central Nervous System.* New York: Raven Press, 1991; 729–39.
4. Tucker T, Ellner JJ. Chronic meningitis. In: Scheld WM, Whitley RJ, Durack DT (eds) *Infections of the Central Nervous System.* New York: Raven Press, 1991; 703–28.
5. Labadie EL, Hamilton RH. Survival improvement in coccidioidal meningitis by high-dose intrathecal amphotericin B. *Arch Intern Med* 1986; **146:** 2013–18.
6. Galgiani JN, Catanzaro A, Cloud GA, Higgs J, et al. Fluconazole therapy for coccidioidal meningitis: the NIAID-*Mycoses* Study Group. *Ann Intern Med* 1993; **119:** 28–35.
7. Sarosi GA, Davies SF. Therapy for fungal infections. *Mayo Clin Proc* 1994; **69:** 1111–17.

78.   Histoplasma capsulatum *meningitis is treated with intravenous amphotericin B*

The recommended therapy of meningitis due to *Histoplasma capsulatum* is intravenous amphotericin B administered in individual doses of at least 50 mg/day in adults and 1 mg/kg/day in children who are less than 50 kg for 6–12 weeks for a total dose of at least 35 mg/kg.[1] Maintenance therapy with 50–80 mg amphotericin B administered weekly or biweekly after a course of induction therapy helps to prevent relapse in individuals infected with human immunodeficiency virus (HIV).[2,3]

References

1. Wheat LJ, Batteiger BE, Sathapatayavongs B. *Histoplasma capsulatum* infections of the central nervous system. *Medicine* 1990; **69:** 244–60.

2. Shaunak S, Cohen J. Clinical management of fungal infection in patients with AIDS. *J Antimicrob Chemo* 1991; **28**(suppl A): 67–81.
3. McKinsey DS, Gupta MR, Riddler SA, Driks MR, Smith DL, Kurtin P. Long-term amphotericin B therapy for disseminated histoplasmosis in patients with acquired immunodeficiency syndrome (AIDS). *Ann Intern Med* 1989; **111**: 655–9.

79. *Immunocompromised patients infected with* Candida, Aspergillus *and Zygomycetes present with stroke-like syndromes and CSF pleocytosis*

Certain fungi, *Candida* spp., *Aspergillus* spp. and the Zygomycetes have a tendency to invade and thrombose cerebral blood vessels. These fungi should be suspected in immunocompromised patients who present with stroke-like syndromes. *Candida* spp. tend to form multiple intraparenchymal micro- or macro-abscesses in the distribution of the middle cerebral artery and mycotic aneurysms. Analysis of the CSF demonstrates an elevated opening pressure, pleocytosis with a predominance of lymphocytes, an elevated protein concentration and a normal or decreased glucose concentration. *Candida* cultures tend to grow rapidly, within 2–4 days, when positive.[1]

Aspergillus spp. infect the CNS in organ transplant recipients typically 1–4 months after transplantation. Several factors increase the risk of an organ transplant recipient developing an infection with *Aspergillus* spp.:

1. immunosuppressive therapy for the treatment of graft rejection;
2. leukopenia;
3. Cytomegalovirus infection.

Aspergillus hyphae tend to invade cerebral blood vessels with subsequent thrombosis, infarction and necrosis. On examination of the CSF, there is an elevated white blood cell count with a predominance of either polymorphonuclear cells or lymphocytes, a normal to elevated protein concentration and a normal glucose concentration. Cerebrospinal fluid smears and cultures are rarely positive. Diagnosis requires culture of tissue.[1,2] Central nervous system infection with Aspergillosis also takes the form of either solitary or multiple brain abscesses.[2]

The Zygomycetes also tend to invade and occlude cerebral blood vessels. The Mucoraceae are in the Zygomycetes class and cause the disease mucormycosis. This is typically an acute fulminant central nervous system infection and tends to occur in immunocompetent diabetic patients with ketoacidosis and in diabetic transplant recipients receiving immunosuppressive agents; therefore, acidosis and hyperglycemia appear to be important predisposing conditions for this infection. Patients who are acidemic from sepsis or other systemic illnesses are also at risk from this infection. The infection tends to originate in the palate or paranasal sinuses and then spreads contiguously through the orbits and paranasal sinuses and into the brain. The infection is often manifest by a black eschar on the palate or nasal mucosa with a blackish purulent discharge from the involved areas (Fig. 79.1). Examination of the CSF demonstrates an elevated opening pressure, a pleocytosis with a predominance of polymorphonuclear cells, a normal glucose concentration and an elevated protein concentration. Diagnosis is made by biopsy of the black eschar.[2]

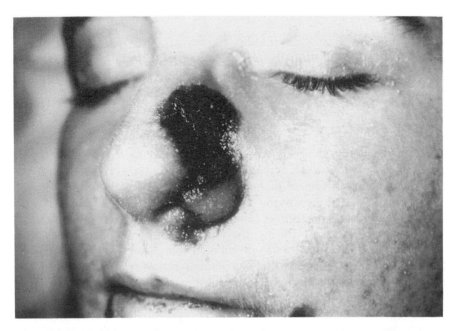

Fig. 79.1 Black eschar of mucormycosis.

With any of the fungal infections, red blood cells or xanthochromia in the CSF may be due to hemorrhagic transformation of an ischemic cerebral infarction or subarachnoid hemorrhage from a ruptured mycotic aneurysm. The laboratory tests that may be helpful in addition to CSF analysis in diagnosing these CNS fungal infections are summarized in Table 72.1 (see maxim 72).

The recommended therapy of a CNS infection due to *Candida*, *Aspergillus* or Zygomycetes is intravenous amphotericin B. *Aspergillus* CNS infections are often fatal and, therefore, high dose intravenous amphotericin B (up to 1.5 mg/kg/day) may be necessary in the treatment of this infection.[1]

References

1. Treseler CB, Sugar AM. Fungal meningitis. *Infect Dis Clin North Amer* 1990; **4**: 789–808.
2. Conti DJ, Rubin RH. Infection of the central nervous system in organ transplant recipients. *Neurol Clin* 1988; **6**: 241–60.

10
Tuberculous Meningitis

---

80. *Tuberculous meningitis is the result of the discharge of tubercle bacilli into the subarachnoid space from subependymal caseous lesions*

Tuberculous meningitis does not develop acutely from hematogenous spread of tubercle bacilli to the meninges. Rich and McCordock[1] are credited with defining the etiology of tuberculous meningitis after performing autopsy examinations of 82 cases of tuberculous meningitis. Isolated miliary tubercles form in the parenchyma of the brain or the meninges during hematogenous dissemination of tubercle bacilli in the course of the primary infection or episodically during the course of chronic tuberculosis from endogenous reactivation of latent tuberculosis elsewhere in the body.[2,3] During the initial stage of infection, small numbers of millet-seed size tubercles are scattered throughout the substance of the brain and meninges. These tubercles tend to enlarge by confluence and growth, and are usually caseating, that is, soft and exudative.[4] The propensity for a caseous lesion to produce meningitis will be determined by its proximity to the subarachnoid space and the rate at which fibrous encapsulation develops due to acquired immune resistance.[3] Subependymal caseous foci may remain quiescent for months or years but then may cause meningitis via discharge of bacilli and tuberculous antigens into the subarachnoid space.[2]

The neurologic complications of tuberculous meningitis are initiated by a hypersensitivity reaction to the discharge of tubercle bacilli and tuberculous antigens into the subarachnoid space. This leads to the production of a thick exudate that fills the basilar cisterns and surrounds the cranial nerves and major blood vessels at the base of the brain, constricting the vessels that comprise the circle of Willis. Within a matter of days, a proliferative arachnoiditis develops. The presence of an inflammatory exudate in the basilar cisterns obstructs the flow of CSF, with resultant obstructive hydrocephalus, and blocks resorption of CSF by the arachnoid granulations as fibrous adhesions develop. Communicating hydrocephalus develops as the resorption of CSF is blocked. Cerebral ischemia and infarction develop as a result of vasculitis due either to a direct invasion of arterial walls by mycobacteria or to compression of the blood vessels at the base of the brain from the adjacent arachnoiditis. Regardless of the etiology, intracranial vasculitis is a major factor contributing to morbidity and mortality from tuberculous meningitis.[3]

References

1. Rich AR, McCordock HA. The pathogenesis of tuberculous meningitis. *Bull Johns Hopkins Hosp* 1933; **52:** 5–37.
2. Molavi A, LeFrock JL. Tuberculous meningitis. *Med Clin North Amer* 1985; **69:** 315–31.
3. Leonard JM, Des Prez RM. Tuberculous meningitis. *Infect Dis Clin North Amer* 1990; **4:** 769–97.
4. Slavin RE, Walsh TJ, Pollack AD. Late generalized tuberculosis: a clinical and pathologic analysis and comparison of 100 cases in the preantibiotic and antibiotic eras. *Medicine* 1980; **59:** 352–66.

81.   *The clinical presentation of tuberculous meningitis is either that of an acute fulminant illness or that of an insidious subacute dementing process*

The clinical presentation of tuberculous meningitis is either that of an acute meningitis syndrome characterized by coma, raised intracranial pressure, seizures and focal neurologic deficits or that of a slowly progressive dementing illness. When the infection presents as an acute meningitis syndrome, characteristic signs and symptoms are headache, malaise, meningismus, papilledema, vomiting, confusion, seizures and cranial nerve deficits. Patients admitted with lethargy or stupor may become comatose in a matter of days. Fever may or may not be present.

Tuberculous meningitis may also present as a slowly progressive dementing illness with memory deficits and personality changes typical of frontal lobe disease, i.e. abulia, and urinary and fecal incontinence. This is the more common presentation of tuberculous meningitis. Cranial nerve deficits and convulsions also occur in the subacute form of tuberculous meningitis.[1] There is often a history of anorexia, cough, night sweats and weight loss days to months prior to the development of symptoms of central nervous system infection (Table 81.1).[2]

A tuberculous encephalopathy is also described. This is a syndrome of convulsions, stupor or coma, involuntary movements, paralysis, and decerebrate spasms or rigidity with or without clinical signs of meningitis or CSF abnormalities of tuberculous meningitis. Pathologically there is either diffuse edema of cerebral white matter with loss of neurons in gray matter, a hemorrhagic leukoencephalopathy, or a post-infectious demyelinating encephalomyelitis. This syndrome has been observed primarily in children with miliary or disseminated tuberculosis.[3,4]

Table 81.1   Signs and symptoms of tuberculous meningitis

Symptoms	Signs
Prodromal	Adenopathy (most commonly cervical)
Anorexia	Adventitious sounds on auscultation
Weight loss	of lungs (apices)
Cough	Choroidal tubercles
Night sweats	Fever (highest in the late afternoon)
CNS	Nuchal rigidity
Headache (worse in recumbancy)	Papilledema
Meningismus	Focal neurologic signs
Altered level of consciousness	Positive tuberculin skin test

Risk factors for tuberculous meningitis include age, alcoholism, infection with human immunodeficiency virus, malnutrition, state of immuno-suppression, drug abuse and homelessness.

References

1. Leonard JM, Des Prez RM. Tuberculous meningitis. *Infect Dis Clin North Amer* 1990; **4:** 769–87.
2. Newton RW. Tuberculous meningitis. *Arch Dis Child* 1994; **70:** 364–6.
3. Udani PM, Dastur DK. Tuberculous encephalopathy with and without meningitis: clinical features and pathologic correlations. *J Neurol Sci* 1970; **10:** 541–61.
4. Molavi A, LeFrock JL. Tuberculous meningitis. *Med Clin North Amer* 1985; **69:** 315–31.

82.   *The absence of pulmonary tuberculosis should not rule out the possibility of tuberculous meningitis*

The diagnosis of tuberculous meningitis is made, and empiric therapy begun, based on a strong clinical suspicion and laboratory data that suggest the diagnosis. The initiation of therapy should not await bacteriologic proof of tubercle bacilli by smear or culture.

Radiographic evidence of pulmonary tuberculosis, specifically hilar adenopathy, is found in 50–90% of cases of tuberculous meningitis in children.[1,2] Zarabi et al.[3] evaluated the chest roentgenogram abnormalities in 180 children with tuberculous meningitis, ranging in age from 1 month to 15 years. Forty-six children (26%) had changes consistent with primary intrathoracic tuberculosis – hilar and/or mediastinal adenopathy, cavities, pneumatoceles and calcification in the hilar area. Twenty-three children (13%) had X-ray findings of disseminated miliary tuberculosis. Fifteen children (8%) showed signs of a miliary pattern with a primary complex, and 15 (8%)

children had areas of intrathoracic calcification. In adults, however, the association of pulmonary lesions and meningitis is not as high, and the absence of pulmonary disease should not rule out a tuberculous etiology for the aseptic meningitis.[2-4]

The classic "Ghon complex" refers to Anton Ghon's observation from autopsy specimens that the primary lesion of tuberculosis is in the lung with secondary infection in the tracheobronchial lymph nodes.[5] In addition to the "primary complex", chest radiographic abnormalities suggestive of pulmonary tuberculosis are hiliar adenopathy, a miliary pattern, upper lobe infiltrate and lobar consolidation. The pathogenesis of central nervous system tuberculosis is discussed in a separate maxim, and it must be borne in mind that CNS disease may develop from caseous foci in organs other than lung with subsequent hematogenous dissemination of virulent tubercle bacilli to the CNS. Mediastinum and abdominal lymph nodes, the adrenal glands, bone and the genitourinary tract are all potential sources of caseous foci which may serve as "seed beds" for the later development of hematogenous dissemination of tubercle bacilli.[6]

The intradermal tuberculin skin test is helpful when positive. The test may, however, be falsely negative even in the absence of immunosuppression and in association with a positive reaction to the common antigens used to determine anergy, i.e. *Candida* and mumps. The tuberculin skin test has been reported to be negative in 50–70% of cases and often becomes positive during the course of therapy.[4,7] The diagnostic studies that should be done for a clinical presentation suggestive of tuberculous meningitis are listed in Table 82.1.

Table 82.1   Diagnostic studies for tuberculous meningitis

---

1. *Tuberculin skin test*

2. *Chest X-ray*
   Hilar adenopathy
   Upper lobe nodular infiltrate
   Miliary pattern

3. *Computed tomography or magnetic resonance imaging*
   Hydrocephalus
   Basilar meningeal enhancement post-contrast
   Cerebral infarction

4. *Cerebrospinal fluid examination*
   Lymphocytic pleocytosis
   Hypoglycorrhacia
   Acid-fast smear and culture

5. *Eye examination for choroidal tubercles*

6. *Sputum and urine smear and culture for acid-fast bacilli*

Communicating or obstructive hydrocephalus, basilar meningeal enhancement following contrast administration and cerebral infarctions are the most frequently reported computed tomography and magnetic resonance imaging abnormalities in tuberculous meningitis. In large series, hydrocephalus is present in 59–76% of cases, meningeal enhancement in 64% of cases and cerebral infarction in 17–53% of cases. Tuberculoma is a less common finding and is present in 10–28% of cases.[8-10] Hydrocephalus is so frequently a complication of tuberculous meningitis in children that, prior to the identification of the tubercle bacillus by Robert Koch in 1882, the diagnostic term most often used for tuberculous meningitis in children was acute hydrocephalus.[11]

References

1. Lee TY, Brown HW. Tuberculous meningitis patients as index cases in the epidemiology of tuberculosis. *Am J Public Health* 1968; **58:** 1901–9.
2. Lincoln EM, Sordillio VR, Davies PA. Tuberculous meningitis in children; a review of 167 untreated and 74 treated patients with special reference to early diagnosis. *J Pediatr* 1960; **57:** 803–23.
3. Zarabi M, Sane S, Girdany BR. The chest roentgenogram in the early diagnosis of tuberculous meningitis in children. *Am J Dis Child* 1971; **121:** 389–92.
4. Molavi A, LeFrock JL. Tuberculous meningitis. *Med Clin North Amer* 1985; **69:** 315–31.
5. Ober WB. Ghon but not forgotten: Anton Ghon and his complex. *Pathol Annual* 1983; **18:** 79–85.
6. Slavin RE, Walsh TJ, Pollack AD. Late generalized tuberculosis: A clinical pathologic analysis and comparison of 100 cases in the preantibiotic and antibiotic eras. *Medicine* 1980; **59:** 352–66.
7. Berenguer J, Moreno S, Laguna F, Vicente T. Tuberculous meningitis in patients infected with the human immunodeficiency virus. *N Engl J Med* 1992; **326:** 668–72.
8. Teoh R, Humphries MJ, Hoare RD, O'Mahony G. Clinical correlation of CT changes in 64 Chinese patients with tuberculous meningitis. *J Neurol* 1989; **236:** 48–51.
9. Kingsley DP, Hendrickse WA, Kendall BE, Swash M, Singh V. Tuberculous meningitis: role of CT in management and prognosis. *J Neurol Neurosurg Psychiatr* 1987; **50:** 30–6.
10. Price HI, Danziger A. Computed tomography in cranial tuberculosis. *Am J Roentgenol* 1978; **130:** 769–71.
11. Meindl JL, Meindl CO. Tuberculous meningitis in the 1830s. *Lancet* 1982; **i**(8271): 554–5.

83.   *Tuberculous meningitis in HIV-infected individuals is very similar to tuberculous meningitis in non-HIV-infected individuals*

The clinical presentation of tuberculous meningitis in patients infected with human immunodeficiency virus (HIV) is very similar to that of tuberculous meningitis in non-HIV-infected patients. There is, however, one very notable exception: that the HIV-infected individual with tuberculous meningitis often has clinical or radiologic evidence of extrameningeal tuberculosis at the time of admission. The presenting symptoms and signs of tuberculous meningitis in 37 HIV-infected patients were fever (89%), headache (59%), altered level of consciousness (43%), malaise (27%) and nausea or vomiting (27%). Twenty-two percent of the HIV-infected individuals had cough compared with 16% of non-HIV-infected individuals.[1] In the majority of the patients with HIV infection in Berenguer's series, analysis of the CSF showed a pleocytosis and hypoglycorrhachia. Acid-fast bacilli were seen on direct smear of CSF from 4 of 18 patients. Chest films demonstrated some type of abnormality suggestive of active tuberculosis in 54% of the HIV-infected individuals. Thoracic and abdominal adenopathy was also a common finding. The tuberculin skin test was positive, producing an area of induration greater than or equal to 10 mm in diameter in 29% of HIV-infected individuals. The CD4 + cell counts were lower than 0.2×10^9/L in 78% of the HIV-infected individuals.[1]

Intracerebral mass lesions are more frequent in HIV-infected individuals than in non-HIV-infected individuals with tuberculous meningitis, occurring in 60% of HIV-infected individuals in one series.[2] The presence of an intra-cerebral mass lesion did not, however, correlate with focal neurologic deficits, altered level of consciousness or mortality in these patients.

References

1. Berenguer J, Moreno S, Laguna F, Vicente T, et al. Tuberculous meningitis in patients infected with the human immunodeficiency virus. *N Engl J Med* 1992; **326:** 668–72.
2. Dube MP, Holtom PD, Larsen RA. Tuberculous meningitis in patients with and without human immunodeficiency virus infection. *Amer J Med* 1992; **93:** 520–4.

84.   *The frequency with which acid-fast bacilli are seen on*
smear of CSF is dependent on both the amount of time devoted
to searching for the organisms and the number of CSF
specimens examined

The classic CSF abnormalities in tuberculous meningitis are:

1. elevated opening pressure;
2. elevated protein concentration in the range of 100–500 mg/dL;
3. white blood cell (WBC) count between 10–500 cells/mm³ with a predominance of lymphocytes;
4. a decreased glucose concentration (Table 84.1).

Table 84.1   Cerebrospinal fluid abnormalities in tuberculous meningitis

1. Increased white blood cell count between 10–500 cells/mm³ with a predominance of lymphocytes

2. Elevated protein concentration in the range of 100 to 500 mg/dL

3. Decreased glucose concentration

4. Cultures positive in 75% of cases requiring 3–6 weeks for growth

5. Decreased chloride concentration

6. Low serum/cerebrospinal fluid bromide ratio

7. Positive tuberculostearic acid assay

At an early stage in the clinical illness, there may be very few WBCs in the CSF, or polymorphonuclear leukocytes may predominate initially with lymphocytes becoming the predominant cell type within 48 hours. A mild elevation in the protein concentration in the CSF with only a few cells present is compatible with tuberculous meningitis. Repeat examination of the CSF will most likely demonstrate a progressive increase in the protein concentration, a progressive decrease in the glucose concentration and a shift to a mononuclear pleocytosis. In addition, there may be a shift in the cell type in the CSF following the initiation of antituberculous therapy from an initial lymphocytic pleocytosis to a predominance of polymorphonuclear leukocytes.[1,2]

The last tube of fluid collected at lumbar puncture is the best tube to send for acid-fast bacilli (AFB) smear. The yield on smear and culture increases, the more samples of CSF that are studied; therefore, three serial CSF samples should be obtained at daily intervals from the lumbar space for smear and culture, or alternatively CSF should be obtained by cisternal puncture for examination. There may be a pellicle in the CSF in tuberculous meningitis or a cobweb-like clot on the surface of the fluid. Acid-fast bacilli can be best demonstrated in a smear of the clot or sediment. If no clot forms, the addition of 2 mL of 95% alcohol results in a heavy protein precipitate which, on centrifuging, draws bacilli to the bottom of the tube. The centrifuged deposit of CSF can then be examined on a glass slide for the bacilli. The amount of time spent searching for the organisms by direct examination of CSF under the microscope is critical to making the diagnosis.[1,3] Positive smears are typically reported in only 10–40% of cases.[4,5]

The most successful technique for identifying the organism requires centrifuging 10–20 mL of CSF at 2500 RPM for 30 minutes and then preparing a thick smear from the pellicle for examination. The smear is then examined for 30 to 90 minutes. Using this technique, organisms have been identified in 91% (91 of 100 cases) of tuberculous meningitis in one series and 85% (122 of 144 cases) in another. This emphasizes the importance of examining the smear for at least 30 minutes.[3,6,7] Even when empiric chemotherapy has been initiated, AFB may be demonstrated on smears of CSF obtained up to 3 days after treatment has begun. Cultures of CSF require 3–6 weeks for growth to be detectable and are positive in approximately 75% of cases of tuberculous meningitis.[1]

The CSF chloride concentration and the bromide partition test have been disappointing in differentiating tuberculous meningitis from other types of lymphocytic meningitis. The CSF chloride concentration may be decreased in tuberculous meningitis to less than 110 mEq/L. However, this is a nonspecific abnormality because the CSF chloride concentration typically decreases as the CSF protein concentration increases, and does not have diagnostic value. The bromide partition test measures the ratio of serum/CSF bromide 24 hours after the oral administration of sodium bromide or the intravenous injection of radioactive bromide.[8] In patients with tuberculous meningitis, the ratio of serum/CSF bromide will be low. A low bromide partition ratio is, however, not specific for tuberculous meningitis and simply represents an increase in the permeability of the blood–CSF barrier.[3]

The enzyme-linked immunosorbent assay (ELISA) has been used in the laboratory to detect *Mycobacterium tuberculosis* antigen and anti-mycobacterial antibodies in spinal fluid. This test, however, is very complex and is primarily useful as a research technique. The determination of CSF adenosine deaminase may be helpful in distinguishing CNS tuberculosis from bacterial meningitis but again is not specific for tuberculous meningitis. The concentration of tuberculostearic acid in spinal fluid has been reported to be a sensitive marker for CNS tuberculosis, but this analysis must be obtained through the Centers for Disease Control as it is not available in most commercial laboratories.

The polymerase chain reaction (PCR) technique for detection of tubercle bacilli DNA in CSF is under development. In the laboratory this technique amplifies the mycobacterial DNA allowing for the identification of the *M. tuberculosis* genome within 24–72 hours.[9,10] The rates of false positive and false negative results and the predictive value of this test are not yet known, and therefore, the PCR assay for the rapid detection of *M. tuberculosis* is not yet recommended for routine clinical use.[11]

References

1. Leonard JM, Des Prez RM. Tuberculous meningitis. *Infect Dis Clin North Amer* 1990; **4**: 769–87.
2. Newton RW. Tuberculous meningitis. *Arch Dis Child* 1994; **70**: 364–6.
3. Molavi A, LeFrock JL. Tuberculous meningitis. *Med Clin North Amer* 1985; **69**: 315–31.
4. Haas FJ, Madhavan T, Quinn EL, et al. Tuberculous meningitis in an urban general hospital. *Arch Intern Med* 1977; **137**: 1518–21.
5. Hinman AR. Tuberculous meningitis at Cleveland Metropolitan General Hospital 1959–1963. *Am Rev Respir Dis* 1967; **95**: 670–3.
6. Stewart SM. The bacteriologic diagnosis of tuberculous meningitis. *J Clin Pathol* 1953; **6**: 241–2.
7. Illingworth RS. Miliary and meningeal tuberculosis: difficulties in diagnosis. *Lancet* 1956; **2**: 646–9.
8. Wiggelinkhuizen J, Mann M. The radioactive bromide partition test in the diagnosis of tuberculous meningitis in children. *J Pediatr* 1980; **97**: 843–7.
9. Yuk-Fong Liu P, Shi ZY, Lau YJ, Hu BS. Rapid diagnosis of tuberculous meningitis by a simplified nested amplification protocol. *Neurology* 1994; **44**: 1161–4.
10. Folgueira L, Delgado R, Palenque E, Noriega A. Polymerase chain reaction for rapid diagnosis of tuberculous meningitis in AIDS patients. *Neurology* 1994; **44**: 1336–8.
11. Macher A, Goosby E. PCR and the misdiagnosis of active tuberculosis. *N Engl J Med* 1995; **332**: 128–9.

85.   *Initiate treatment of tuberculous meningitis with three-drug therapy*

A combination of three antituberculous drugs is recommended for the treatment of tuberculous meningitis in adults. Treatment should be initiated as follows:

1. isoniazid 5 mg/kg/day, maximum dose 300 mg/day;
2. rifampin 10 mg/kg/day, maximum dose 600 mg/day; and
3. pyrazinamide 15–30 mg/kg/day, maximum dose 2 g/day (Table 85.1).

Pyridoxine 50 mg/day is given with isoniazid to prevent the development of a peripheral neuropathy. In cases where antimicrobial resistance is suspected, ethambutol 15–20 mg/kg/day can be used in the initial regimen. If the clinical response is fairly good, pyrazinamide and ethambutol can be discontinued after 8 weeks and isoniazid and rifampin continued alone for the remaining 9–12 months.[1,2]

In individuals infected with the human immunodeficiency virus (HIV), the recommended regimen is:

1. isoniazid 10–15 mg/kg/day;
2. rifampin 10–15 mg/kg/day; and
3. either ethambutol 25 mg/kg/day or pyrazinamide 20–30 mg/kg/day, and either streptomycin, rifabutin or clofazimine.

Table 85.1   Antituberculous chemotherapy

Drug	Dosage	
	Children	Adults
Isoniazid	10 mg/kg/day once daily	300 mg/day
Rifampin	10 mg/kg/day	10 mg/kg/day
Ethambutol	15–25 mg/kg/day in divided doses	15–25 mg/kg/day in divided doses
Pyrazinamide	30 mg/kg/day in divided doses	30 mg/kg/day in divided doses
Streptomycin	20–40 mg/kg/day once daily	1 g once daily

Source: Committee on Infectious Diseases. Chemotherapy for tuberculosis in infants and children. *Pediatrics* 1992; **89:** 161–4.

Treatment is continued for at least 6–9 months and at least 6 months beyond the demonstration of negative cultures.[2]

For tuberculous meningitis in children, the American Academy of Pediatrics recommends a 12-month regimen using the following antibiotics until drug susceptibility is known:

1. isoniazid 10–15 mg/kg/day, maximum daily dose 300 mg;
2. rifampin 10–20 mg/kg/day, maximum daily dose 600 mg;
3. pyrazinamide 20–40 mg/kg/day, maximum daily dose 2 g;
4. streptomycin 20–40 mg/kg/day.

The combination of isoniazid, rifampin, pyrazinamide and streptomycin is continued for 2 months, followed by isoniazid and rifampin administered daily or twice weekly under medical supervision for 10 months. When isoniazid is administered twice weekly the dose is 20–40 mg/kg/dose and when rifampin is administered twice weekly the dose is 10–20 mg/kg/dose. The American Academy of Pediatrics recommends that liver function be monitored during the first several months of treatment. The Academy also recommends that the administration of corticosteroids be considered in cases of tuberculous meningitis.[3] Dexamethasone may be administered in a dose of 0.3–0.5 mg/kg/day in the first week of treatment followed by prednisone

2 mg/kg/day, tapered gradually over 3–4 weeks.[4]

The major adverse effect of ethambutol is optic neuropathy. The incidence of this side effect is more common at higher doses of the drug; therefore therapy can be initiated at 25 mg/kg/day then reduced to 15 mg/kg/day after a few months when the decision is made to continue this agent. The major adverse effects of the antituberculous agents are listed in Table 85.2.

Table 85.2   Major adverse effects of antituberculous agents

Drug	Adverse effects
Isoniazid	Hepatic toxicity Peripheral neuropathy (can be prevented with pyridoxine) Phenytoin toxicity
Rifampin	Hepatic toxicity Interstitial nephritis
Ethambutol	Optic neuropathy
Pyrazinamide	Hepatic toxicity Arthralgias with hyperuricemia
Streptomycin	Vestibular toxicity

Immunization with the BCG (bacillus of Calmette and Guerin) vaccine is recommended only for tuberculin skin-test negative children who are at risk of exposure to tuberculosis. It is not recommended in individuals with the human immunodeficiency virus because of the potential to develop disseminated *Mycobacterium bovis* infection.[2]

References

1. Snider DE, Rieder HL, Combs D, Bloch AB, Hayden CH, et al. Tuberculosis in children. *Pediatr Infect Dis J* 1988; **7**: 271–8.
2. Holdiness MR. Management of tuberculosis meningitis. *Drugs* 1990; **39**(2): 224–33.
3. Committee on Infectious Diseases. Chemotherapy for tuberculosis in infants and children. *Pediatrics* 1992; **89**: 161–4.
4. Jacobs RF, Sunakorn P, Chotpitayasunonah T, Pope S, Kelleher K. Intensive short course chemotherapy for tuberculous meningitis. *Pediatr Infect Dis J* 1992; **11**: 194–8.

86.   There are limited indications for the use of corticosteroids in tuberculous meningitis

The rationale and indications for the use of corticosteroids in tuberculous meningitis are similar to those for bacterial meningitis. In experimental models of bacterial meningitis, dexamethasone decreases brain edema, decreases CSF outflow resistance, decreases the production of inflammatory cytokines, decreases the number of leukocytes, and therefore the inflammatory mass in the subarachnoid space, and minimizes the damage to the blood–brain barrier. In patients with acute tuberculous meningitis with altered consciousness and raised intracranial pressure, corticosteroids may be beneficial, as the pathophysiology of coma and raised intracranial pressure is similar in both diseases. In patients with a subacute presentation of meningitis, corticosteroids are probably of little benefit as cerebral edema and increased intracranial pressure are not the etiology of the neurologic complications.

The main argument against using corticosteroids is that they decrease meningeal inflammation and meningeal inflammation is necessary to ensure the penetration of antituberculous drugs into the subarachnoid space. Rifampin, for example, crosses the blood–brain barrier adequately only when inflammation is present. Isoniazid and pyrazinamide, on the other hand, diffuse very well into the CSF through normal and inflamed meninges. Concomitant treatment with corticosteroids would not be expected to decrease the CSF penetration of isoniazid or pyrazinamide. In a clinical trial in which 8 patients were treated with isoniazid, rifampin, streptomycin and pyrazinamide in combination and corticosteroids (dexamethasone 5 mg intravenously every 6 hours during the first week followed by oral prednisolone, 60 mg daily), the use of corticosteroids did not reduce the CSF concentrations of any of the antituberculous drugs.[1]

In one of the largest clinical trials reported to date, 280 patients with a clinical presentation of tuberculous meningitis were treated with either dexamethasone (12 mg/day to adults and 8 mg/day to children, intramuscularly) and antituberculous chemotherapy or antituberculous chemotherapy alone. In 160 patients, *Mycobacterium tuberculosis* was cultured from the CSF. In the remaining 120 patients, the diagnosis was a clinical diagnosis only. Most of the patients (96%) were either drowsy or comatose at the time of admission. The results of this clinical trial demonstrated a significant reduction in mortality, neurologic complications, and a significantly more rapid normalization of the CSF white blood cell count, protein and glucose concentrations, in the patients treated with dexamethasone plus antituberculous chemotherapy than in the patients treated with antituberculous chemotherapy alone.[2] These same investigators had previously observed a beneficial effect of dexamethasone in reducing ocular complications in patients with tuberculous meningitis.[3]

Dexamethasone is recommended in cases of tuberculous meningitis in which one of the following complications has developed:

1. altered consciousness;
2. papilledema;
3. focal neurologic deficit; and/or
4. CSF opening pressure greater than 300 mmH$_2$O.[4]

References

1. Kaojarern S, Supmonchai K, Phuapradit P, Mokkhavesa C, Krittiyanunt S. Effects of steroids on cerebrospinal fluid penetration of antituberculous drugs in tuberculous meningitis. *Clin Pharmacol Ther* 1991; **49:** 6–12.
2. Girgis NI, Farid Z, Kilpatrick ME, Sultan Y, Mikhail IA. Dexamethasone adjunctive treatment for tuberculous meningitis. *Pediatr Infect Dis J* 1991; **10:** 179–83.
3. Girgis NI, Farid Z, Hanna LS, Yassin MW, Wallace CK. The use of dexamethasone in preventing ocular complications in tuberculous meningitis. *Trans Roy Soc Trop Med Hyg* 1983; **77:** 658–9.
4. Molavi A, LeFrock JL. Tuberculous meningitis. *Med Clin North Amer* 1985; **69:** 315–31.

87.   *The most important prognostic factor in tuberculous meningitis is the level of consciousness at the initiation of therapy*

The most important prognostic factor that is reported repeatedly in cases of tuberculous meningitis is the level of consciousness at the initiation of therapy. The greater the alteration in mental status, the worse the outcome. The mortality rate of patients who are comatose prior to the initiation of therapy is 50–70%.[1] Other factors that may adversely affect outcome include:

1. age (the mortality rate is highest in the very young and the very old);
2. malnutrition;
3. the presence of miliary disease;
4. the presence of an underlying debilitating disease such as alcoholism;
5. hydrocephalus;
6. cerebrovascular complications;
7. low CSF glucose concentration;
8. elevated CSF protein concentration.[1,2]

In patients with the human immunodeficiency virus infection, the duration of illness prior to the institution of therapy and a low total CD4 + cell count are the most significant prognostic indicators.[3]

References

1. Molavi A, LeFrock JL. Tuberculous meningitis. *Med Clin North Amer* 1985; **69:** 315–31.
2. Delage G, Dusseault TM. Tuberculous meningitis in children: a retrospective study of 79 patients, with an analysis of prognostic factors. *Can Med Assoc J* 1979; **120:** 305–9.
3. Berenguer J, Moreno S, Laguna S, Vicente T, et al. Tuberculous meningitis in patients infected with the human immunodeficiency virus. *N Engl J Med* 1992; **326:** 668–72.

11
Syphilitic Meningitis

88. *The most common presentation of neurosyphilis today is syphilitic meningitis and meningovascular syphilis*

Six neurosyphilitic syndromes are described: asymptomatic neurosyphilis, acute syphilitic meningitis, meningovascular syphilis, parenchymatous neurosyphilis (dementia paralytica and/or tabes dorsalis), CNS gummata, and congenital neurosyphilis.[1] In the preantibiotic era, tabes dorsalis was the most common form of neurosyphilis. Over the past decade, an increasing number of cases of early neurosyphilis (asymptomatic or symptomatic syphilitic meningitis and vasculitis) and syphilitic eye disease have been reported. The increasing number of cases of early neurosyphilis are occurring in individuals also infected with the human immunodeficiency virus (HIV).[2-4] The various neurosyphilitic syndromes are described below.

Asymptomatic neurosyphilis

The examination of the CSF is abnormal in a syphilis patient without clinical signs or symptoms of neurologic involvement. There is typically an elevated CSF protein concentration, a mild mononuclear pleocytosis and a positive venereal disease research laboratory (VDRL) test.[1,2]

Acute syphilitic meningitis

This form of neurosyphilis was first described by H. Houston Merritt in 1935.[5] The most common symptoms are headache, nausea and vomiting. There is usually evidence of meningeal irritation, i.e. stiffness of the neck and Kernig's sign. In Merritt's review, papilledema was frequently present, due to acute hydrocephalus with increased intracranial pressure. There also may be evidence of cranial nerve palsies involving cranial nerves III, VI, VII and VIII. The meningeal symptoms typically develop within 1 year of the initial infection, most often within 3–7 months after the appearance of the chancre. In 10% of cases, the development of neurologic signs and symptoms coincides with the papulosquamous rash of secondary syphilis. Examination of the CSF in cases of syphilitic meningitis reveals an increased opening pressure, a mononuclear pleocytosis, an elevated protein concentration and a positive VDRL test. A nonreactive CSF–VDRL test does not rule out neurosyphilis. A reactive CSF–VDRL test virtually confirms the diagnosis of neurosyphilis except when the CSF is blood-tinged.[1,4,5] A false-positive CSF–VDRL test may be obtained when the CSF is contaminated with visible amounts of blood.[6]

Meningovascular syphilis

This stage is defined by the appearance of focal neurologic signs, due to an inflammatory, obliterative endarteritis involving small and medium-sized arteries. The clinical presentation may be that of stroke due to brain infarction or intracerebral hemorrhage. The diagnosis is made by cerebral angiography which demonstrates concentric narrowing of the intradural vessels or occlusion of the proximal branches of the anterior and middle cerebral arteries. Lumbar puncture should be performed cautiously in these patients as brain infarction or intracerebral hemorrhage may be associated with massive cerebral edema.[7,8] The vascular supply to the spinal cord may be similarly affected.

Tabes dorsalis

The signs and symptoms of tabes dorsalis are due to neuronal degeneration and infiltration of inflammatory cells in the dorsal columns and posterior spinal nerve roots of the spinal cord. They include episodic lancinating pain in the lower extremities, progressive ataxia, loss of vibration and position sense, areflexia, disturbances of micturition (from the deafferentated bladder), impotence and optic atrophy. The ataxia is a typical "sensory ataxia" with a broad-based, foot-slapping gait. The classic pupillary abnormality is the Argyll Robertson pupil. There is loss of the pupillary reaction to light with preservation of pupillary constriction to accommodation.[1,2,7,8] This form of neurosyphilis has the longest latent period between primary infection and onset of symptoms, with the development of symptoms typically 20–30 years after primary infection.

Dementia paralytica

This stage of neurosyphilis is characterized by a slow deterioration in cognitive functioning. Initially there are signs of forgetfulness and personality changes, making a distinction from Alzheimer's disease difficult. As the disease progresses, there is impaired memory, loss of insight and judgment, dysphasia, loss of appendicular strength, pupillary abnormalities, and loss of bowel and bladder control. The syndrome of dementia paralytica most often occurs 10–30 years following the primary infection.[1,8] Examination of the CSF at this stage demonstrates one or a combination of the following: a positive VDRL test, lymphocytic pleocytosis, and/or an elevated protein concentration. The serum VDRL test may be negative in 25% of patients; however specific treponemal tests such as the fluorescent treponemal antibody absorption test and the microhemagglutination–*Treponema pallidum* test should be reactive.[1]

Gummatous neurosyphilis

Intracranial gummata were extremely rare in Houston Merritt's days and are extremely rare today. When they do occur, they are most often found in the basilar cisterns or encasing the cranial nerves. They are easily identified by a computed tomography scan or magnetic resonance imaging. They manifest as space occupying lesions or cranial nerve palsies.[7]

References

1. Johnson RA, White M. Syphilis in the 1990s: cutaneous and neurologic manifestations. *Semin Neurol* 1992; **12:** 287–98.
2. Marra CM. Syphilis and human immunodeficiency virus infection. *Semin Neurol* 1992; **12:** 43–50.
3. Johns DR, Tierney M, Felsenstein D. Alteration in the natural history of neurosyphilis by concurrent infection with the human immunodeficiency virus. *N Engl J Med* 1987; **316:** 1569–72.
4. Katz DA, Berger JR. Neurosyphilis in acquired immunodeficiency syndrome. *Arch Neurol* 1989; **46:** 895–8.
5. Merritt HH, Moore M. Acute syphilitic meningitis. *Medicine* 1935; **14:** 119–83.
6. Davis LE, Sperry S. The CSF–FTA test and the significance of blood contamination. *Ann Neurol* 1979; **6:** 68–9.
7. Prange HW, Bleck TP. Neurosyphilis. In: Hacke W (ed.), *NeuroCritical Care*. Berlin: Springer-Verlag, 1994; 418–27.
8. Roos KL. Neurosyphilis. *Semin Neurol* 1992; **12:** 209–12.

89.   *The FTA–ABS test and the MHA–TP test remain positive for life; the VDRL titer falls after treatment*

The serologic tests for syphilis can be grouped into two categories: treponemal tests, which detect specific antibodies against *Treponema pallidum*, and nontreponemal tests which detect antibodies to lipids found on the membranes of *T. pallidum* using cardiolipin–lecithin–cholesterol antigens. The treponemal tests in routine use include the fluorescent treponemal antibody absorption test (FTA–ABS) and the microhemagglutination–*T. pallidum* test (MHA–TP). The nontreponemal tests in routine use today include the venereal disease research laboratory test (VDRL) and the rapid plasma reagin test (RPR). The treponemal tests become positive earlier in the course of infection and are more specific than the nontreponemal tests. Treponemal tests become positive 3–4 weeks after inoculation. Nontreponemal tests become positive 5–6 weeks after inoculation. The FTA–ABS test is the first serologic test to become positive. The FTA–ABS test may be positive in about 25% of patients with either a negative VDRL or MHA–TP.

The treponemal tests are nonquantitative; they are either positive or negative. The VDRL test may be quantitated by serial dilutions of serum, and the titer is reported as the greatest serum dilution that produces a positive result. The VDRL titer rises rapidly and peaks during the first year of infection after which it gradually declines, reaching low levels in late syphilis and eventually becoming nonreactive in about 25% of untreated patients. After adequate treatment of syphilis, the titer falls at a rate that is related to the duration of infection before treatment was initiated.

The causes of biological false-positive VDRL and FTA–ABS tests are listed in Table 89.1.[1,2]

Table 89.1   False-positive serologic tests for syphilis

1. *False-positive fluorescent treponemal antibody absorption (FTA–ABS) test*
   Technical error
   Lyme borreliosis
   Genital herpes simplex
   Lupus erythematosus
   Scleroderma
   Mixed connective tissue disease
   Cirrhosis
   Nonvenereal treponematoses
2. *Transient (<6 months) false-positive venereal disease research laboratory (VDRL) test*
   Mycoplasma pneumoniae
   Enterovirus infection
   Infectious mononucleosis
   Tuberculosis
   Viral pneumonia
   Leptospirosis
   Measles
   Mumps
3. *Chronic false-positive VDRL test (lasting longer than 6 months)*
   Systemic lupus erythematosus and other connective tissue disorders
   Intravenous drug use
   Rheumatoid arthritis
   Reticuloendothelial malignancy
   Age (elderly persons)
   Hashimoto's thyroiditis

In a patient suspected of having neurosyphilis, a serologic test for syphilis is performed initially. The FTA–ABS, MHA–TP, and VDRL are reported to have a sensitivity of 100% in cases of untreated secondary syphilis. In symptomatic late syphilis, the VDRL test is reported to have a sensitivity of 70%, the MHA–TP a sensitivity of 94–100% and the FTA–ABS a sensitivity of 100%.[3-6] It is important to note that because the VDRL test may become nonreactive in later stages of syphilis, only about 70% of patients with neurosyphilis have a positive VDRL test. Patients suspected of having neurosyphilis should be screened for the disease with either the FTA–ABS test or the MHA–TP test. Biological false-positive serologic tests have been previously attributed to pregnancy; however, it is recommended that the detection of a positive serologic test in a pregnant woman be treated as a true positive test. Most false-positive VDRL tests have a low titer of 1:8 or less. Ten percent of elderly individuals aged 80 or older have a low titer false-positive VDRL test.

The specificity and sensitivity of syphilis serologic tests are not the same in individuals infected with human immunodeficiency virus 1 (HIV-1) as in non-HIV-infected individuals. The non-treponemal tests for syphilis have been shown to be falsely negative in at least one HIV-1-infected patient. Screening for syphilis in HIV-1-infected individuals should be performed by the serum FTA–ABS test. There are, however, antecdotal reports of false-negative tests in HIV-1-infected individuals with secondary, latent and tertiary syphilis. In addition, there is a loss of reactivity to the treponemal tests in individuals infected with HIV-1. The sensitivity of these tests in identifying prior episodes of syphilis in individuals with symptomatic HIV infection has been reported to be as low as 62%. The loss of treponemal test reactivity increases as immune dysfunction progresses in acquired immune deficiency syndrome, and is particularly low in association with a T_4-lymphocyte count below 200/mm^3.[7-10]

References

1. Johnson RA, White M. Syphilis in the 1990s: cutaneous and neurologic manifestations. *Semin Neurol* 1992; **12:** 287–98.
2. Roos KL. Neurosyphilis. *Semin Neurol* 1992; **12:** 209–12.
3. Hart G. Syphilis tests in diagnostic and therapeutic decision making. *Ann Intern Med* 1986; **104:** 368–76.
4. Larsen SA, Hambie EA, Pettit DP, Perryman MW, Kraus SJ. Specificity, sensitivity, and reproducibility among the fluorescent treponemal antibody-absorption test, the microhemagglutination assay for *Treponema pallidum* antibodies, and the hemagglutination treponemal test for syphilis. *J Clin Microbiol* 1981; **14:** 441–5.
5. Deacon WE, Lucas JB, Price EB. Fluorescent treponemal antibody-absorption (FTA–ABS) test for syphilis. *JAMA* 1966; **198:** 624–8.
6. Lesinski J, Krach J, Kadziewicz E. Specificity, sensitivity, and diagnostic value of the TPHA test. *Br J Vener Dis* 1974; **50:** 334–40.
7. Haas JS, Bolan G, Larsen SA, Clement MJ, Bacchetti P, Moss AR. Sensitivity of treponemal tests for detecting prior treated syphilis during human immunodeficiency virus infection. *J Infect Dis* 1990; **162:** 862–6.
8. Hicks CB, Benson PM, Lupton GP, Tramont EC. Seronegative secondary syphilis

in a patient infected with human immunodeficiency virus (HIV) with Kaposi sarcoma. *Ann Intern Med* 1987; **107:** 492–5.

9. Johnson PDR, Graves SR, Stewart L, Warren R, Dwyer B, Lucas CR. Specific syphilis serologic tests may become negative in HIV infection. *AIDS* 1991; **5:** 419–23.

10. Katz DA, Berger JR. Neurosyphilis in acquired immunodeficiency syndrome. *Arch Neurol* 1989; **46:** 895–8.

90.   *Screening for neurosyphilis should include a combination of nontreponemal and treponemal serum serologic tests and an examination of the CSF*

The following steps should be followed in individuals suspected of having neurosyphilis:

1. Serum venereal disease research laboratory (VDRL) test or rapid plasma reagin (RPR) test.
2. Serum fluorescent treponemal antibody absorption test (FTA–ABS) or *Treponema pallidum* hemagglutination assay (TPHA).
3. Examination of the CSF for the following:
    a. a reactive VDRL
    b. lymphocytic pleocytosis
    c. elevated protein concentration.

The diagnosis of neurosyphilis is made in the presence of a reactive nontreponemal and treponemal serologic test (Table 90.1),[1,2] with either neurologic manifestations consistent with neurosyphilis and/or a CSF examination suggestive of neurosyphilis. The latter is suggestive of neurosyphilis with either a reactive VDRL test or a lymphocytic pleocytosis and an elevated protein concentration. The CSF VDRL may be nonreactive in 30–57% of samples of CSF from patients with neurosyphilis.[3,4]

Table 90.1   Serologic tests for syphilis

Treponemal tests
Detect specific antibody to *Treponema pallidum* antigen
    1. FTA–ABS: fluorescent treponemal antibody absorption test
    2. MHA–TP: microhemagglutination assay for *Treponema pallidum*
Non-treponemal tests
Detect antibodies to lipids found on the membranes of *T. pallidum*, using antigens such as cardiolipin, lecithin or cholesterol
    1. VDRL: venereal disease research laboratory test
    2. RPR: rapid plasma reagin test

In Europe, treponemal tests (such as the TPHA) are used routinely on CSF to make a diagnosis of neurosyphilis. These tests on CSF are, however, not available in the United States. When the TPHA on CSF is available, a TPHA index can be determined as follows:

$$\text{ITpA index} = \frac{\text{TPHA}_{CSF}/\text{Total IgG}_{CSF}}{\text{TPHA}_{serum}/\text{Total IgG}_{serum}}$$

A value >2.0 confirms the diagnosis of neurosyphilis. The ITpA (intrathecally produced *T. pallidum*-specific antibodies) index remains positive throughout life and cannot be interpreted as a criterion of activity in patients who have been treated for neurosyphilis.[3,5] A polymerase chain reaction (PCR) to detect *T. pallidum* in CSF is also available. The results in some clinical trials have suggested, however, that the PCR using CSF is not a sensitive method for the diagnosis of neurosyphilis.[6]

In individuals infected with human immunodeficiency virus (HIV) with symptomatic early neurosyphilis (meningitis, cranial-nerve abnormalities or stroke) the diagnosis of neurosyphilis can be made by the above recommendations. The majority of these patients have positive serum serologic tests for syphilis (RPR or VDRL), a positive CSF VDRL test and a mild CSF pleocytosis or elevated protein concentration.[7] The serum RPR titers are often higher in individuals with early HIV and syphilis than in those without HIV.[8] However, in individuals with advanced HIV-related illness, the serum nontreponemal and treponemal tests may be negative even in instances of well-documented secondary, ocular or neurosyphilis.[9,10]

References

1. Johnson RA, White M. Syphilis in the 1990s: cutaneous and neurologic manifestations. *Semin Neurol* 1992; **12**: 287–98.
2. Hart G. Syphilis tests in diagnostic and therapeutic decision making. *Ann Intern Med* 1986; **104**: 368–76.
3. Luger A, Schmidt BL, Steyrer K, Schonwald E. Diagnosis of neurosyphilis by examination of the cerebrospinal fluid. *Br J Vener Dis* 1981; **57**: 232–7.
4. Dans PE, Cafferty L, Otter SE, Johnson RJ. Inappropriate use of the cerebrospinal fluid Venereal Disease Research Laboratory (VDRL) test to exclude neurosyphilis. *Ann Intern Med* 1986; **104**: 86–9.
5. Prange HW, Bleck TP. Neurosyphilis. In: Hacke W (ed.), *NeuroCritical Care*. Berlin: Springer-Verlag, 1994; 418–27.
6. Gordon SM, Eaton ME, George R, et al. The response of symptomatic neurosyphilis to high-dose intravenous penicillin G in patients with human immunodeficiency virus infection. *N Engl J Med* 1994; **331**: 1469–72.
7. Matlow AG, Rachlis AR. Syphilis serology in human immunodeficiency virus-infected patients with symptomatic neurosyphilis: case report and review. *Rev Infect Dis* 1990; **12**: 703–7.
8. Hutchinson CM, Rompalo AM, Reichart CA, Hook EW III. Characteristics of syphilis patients attending Baltimore STD Clinics: multiple high risk subgroups and interactions with human immunodeficiency virus infection. *Arch Intern Med* 1991; **151**: 511–16.

9. Marra CM. Syphilis and human immunodeficiency virus infection. *Semin Neurol* 1992; **12:** 43–50.
10. Hicks CB, Benson PM, Lupton GP, Tramont EC. Seronegative secondary syphilis in a patient infected with the human immunodeficiency virus (HIV) with Kaposi sarcoma: a diagnostic dilemma. *Ann Intern Med* 1987; **107:** 492–5.

91.   *Primary, secondary and latent syphilis are treated with benzathine penicillin; neurosyphilis is treated with intravenous aqueous penicillin G*

The Centers for Disease Control recommend intravenous aqueous crystalline penicillin G, 2–4 million units every 4 hours for 10–14 days for treatment of neurosyphilis. An alternate regimen is procaine penicillin, 2.4 million units intramuscularly daily with probenecid, 500 mg orally four times daily, both for 10–14 days. The latter therapy may not reliably achieve treponemicidal penicillin levels within the CSF, though well-documented instances of failure of this therapy have not been reported.[1–3]

For the treatment of primary, secondary and early latent syphilis of less than 1 year's duration, the Centers for Disease Control recommend the use of benzathine penicillin G, 2.4 million units intramuscularly in one dose. For penicillin-allergic patients, doxycycline 100 mg orally twice daily for 2 weeks can be used. For treatment of latent syphilis of more than 1 year's duration, benzathine penicillin G is administered in three doses of 2.4 million units per dose intramuscularly given 1 week apart for 3 consecutive weeks.[3] In recent years, 1.0 g of ceftriaxone administered intramuscularly has been investigated; however, preliminary data show a 25% failure rate of the ceftriaxone regimen for asymptomatic neurosyphilis.[1,4]

References

1. Marra CM. Syphilis and human immunodeficiency virus infection. *Semin Neurol* 1992; **12:** 43–50.
2. van der Valk PGM, Kraai EJ, van Voorst Vader PC, et al. Penicillin concentrations in cerebrospinal fluid (CSF) during repository treatment regimen for syphilis. *Genitourin Med* 1988; **64:** 223–5.
3. Johnson RA, White M. Syphilis in the 1990s: cutaneous and neurologic manifestations. *Semin Neurol* 1992; **12:** 287–98.
4. Dowell ME, Ross PG, Cate TR, et al. Ceftriaxone therapy for HIV-infected persons with late latent syphilis or asymptomatic neurosyphilis. (Abstract) *Abstracts of the 1991 Interscience Conference on Antimicrobial Agents Chemotherapy.* Washington DC: American Society for Microbiology, 1991; 148.

92. *The Jarisch–Herxheimer reaction may occur when antibiotic therapy is initiated for the treatment of syphilitic meningitis*

The Jarisch–Herxheimer reaction most often occurs within 24 hours after the initiation of antimicrobial treatment for syphilis, and is an acute febrile reaction associated with chills, arterial hypotension, tachycardia, nausea, headaches, myalgia and worsening of CNS symptomatology. The incidence of this reaction is highest in the early stages of syphilis and fairly rare in cases of neurosyphilis. The pathogenic mechanism is an immunologic reaction to antigen or pyrogen release from dead spirochetes. Patients should be informed that the reaction may occur and, in severe cases, admission to an intensive care unit may be indicated. Steroid therapy may be beneficial.[1,2]

References

1. Johnson RA, White M. Syphilis in the 1990s: cutaneous and neurologic manifestations. *Semin Neurol* 1992; **12**: 287–98.
2. Prange HW, Bleck TP. Neurosyphilis. In: Hacke W (ed.), *NeuroCritical Care*. Berlin: Springer-Verlag, 1994; 418–27.

93. *Benzathine penicillin G may not be adequate therapy for primary or secondary syphilis in individuals also infected with HIV*

The use of benzathine penicillin G for early syphilis may not be effective in patients with human immunodeficiency virus (HIV) infection. These patients often have clinical or laboratory evidence of infection in the CNS despite therapy for early syphilis with doses of benzathine penicillin G as high as 7.2 million units.[1] This group of patients may also have asymptomatic neurosyphilis at the time they are evaluated and treated for primary or secondary syphilis. This has led to the recommendation that all patients who are seropositive for HIV and syphilis have a CSF examination to rule out neurosyphilis regardless of the duration of syphilis or the presence of neurologic signs and symptoms.[2]

In addition to reports of relapse of disease in the CNS despite therapy for early syphilis that met or exceeded current recommendations, there are also reports of failure of intravenous aqueous penicillin G, 18–24 million units/day for 10 days, to treat neurosyphilis in HIV-infected individuals.[1] Re-examination of CSF should be part of the follow-up for therapy of neurosyphilis in this patient population. The interpretation of CSF abnormalities for therapeutic decisions is, however, difficult. In patients without concurrent HIV infection, the initial CSF pleocytosis will resolve 6 months after penicillin therapy in 80% of patients, and 1 year after therapy in 90%. Serial venereal disease research laboratory (VDRL) test titers on CSF should decrease following treatment, but it may take years for the CSF to become nonreactive.[1,3,4] The persistence of a CSF pleocytosis, a rising CSF VDRL titer, or signs and symptoms of neurosyphilis, would be an indication to retreat for neurosyphilis.

It is not clear why antibiotic treatment fails in HIV-infected individuals or why the natural history of neurosyphilis appears to be altered in individuals coinfected with HIV. In the era before HIV infection, the mean length of time to presentation of neurosyphilis following primary syphilis with no therapy at all, was at least 15 years. The typical presentation of neurosyphilis was dementia paralytica and/or tabes dorsalis. In contrast, in individuals infected with HIV, the syndromes of early neurosyphilis are common, including meningitis, cranial nerve abnormalities and stroke, and are typically seen less than 1 year after the onset of infection. In the era before HIV infection, a case of neurosyphilis after treatment for early syphilis with benzathine penicillin G was rare. HIV-infected individuals have an accelerated progression to early neurosyphilis and, in these individuals, conventional therapy for primary and secondary syphilis is more often ineffective, and there is no certain cure for neurosyphilis in HIV-infected individuals.[5,6]

References

1. Gordon SM, Eaton ME, George R, et al. The response of symptomatic neurosyphilis to high-dose intravenous penicillin G in patients with human immunodeficiency virus infection. *N Engl J Med* 1994; **331**: 1469–72.
2. Johns DR, Tierney M, Felsenstein D. Alteration in the natural history of neurosyphilis by concurrent infection with the human immunodeficiency virus. *N Engl J Med* 1987; **316**: 1569–72.
3. Hahn RD, Cutler JC, Curtis AC, et al. Penicillin treatment of asymptomatic central nervous system syphilis. II. Results of therapy as measured by laboratory findings. *Arch Dermatol* 1956; **74**: 367–77.
4. Dattner B, Thomas EW, De Mello L. Criteria for the management of neurosyphilis. *Am J Med* 1951; **10**: 463–7.
5. Musher DM. Syphilis, neurosyphilis, penicillin and AIDS. *J Infect Dis* 1991; **163**: 1201–6.
6. Musher DM, Baughn RE. Neurosyphilis in HIV-infected persons. *N Engl J Med* 1994; **331**: 1516–17.

94.   *A lumbar puncture to rule out neurosyphilis is indicated in patients with slowly progressive dementing illnesses and all HIV-infected patients with primary syphilis*

As has been described in maxim 88 on the neurosyphilitic syndromes, the initial clinical manifestation of dementia paralytica is a slow deterioration in cognitive functioning very similar to that which occurs in Alzheimer's disease. These patients should have a lumbar puncture to rule out a treatable form of dementia, neurosyphilis. In addition, all human immunodeficiency virus (HIV)-infected patients with syphilis should have a CSF examination. The early neurosyphilitic syndromes, asymptomatic and syphilitic meningitis, are more common than the late neurosyphilitic syndromes in patients with HIV infection. Results of the CSF evaluation in these patients can guide the choice of treatment. Patients infected with HIV with a CSF pleocytosis or a reactive CSF venereal disease research laboratory (VDRL) test can be assumed to have asymptomatic neurosyphilis and be treated with a penicillin regimen that is recommended for neurosyphilis. Patients infected with HIV and syphilis but a normal CSF can be treated with the recommended dose of benzathine penicillin for primary, secondary or latent syphilis.[1,2]

References

1. Johnson RA, White M. Syphilis in the 1990s: cutaneous and neurologic mani-festations. *Semin Neurol* 1992; **12:** 287–98.
2. Marra CM. Syphilis and human immunodeficiency virus infection. *Semin Neurol* 1992; **12:** 43–50.

12
Carcinomatous Meningitis

95. *By definition, the dissemination of malignant cells throughout the leptomeninges is referred to as neoplastic or carcinomatous meningitis, specifically as carcinomatous meningitis when leptomeningeal metastases develop from solid tumors, and lymphomatous or leukemic meningitis when the meninges are seeded during the course of these diseases*

Carcinomatous meningitis was first described by Eberth[1] in 1870, but the metastatic nature of the disease was not appreciated, and it was attributed to an unassociated "endothelioma" of the meninges. Individual case reports were described by Oppenheim[2] in 1888 and Siefert[3] in 1902, but the term "meningeal carcinomatosis" was first used by Beerman[4] in 1912 to describe a case of diffuse leptomeningeal metastasis by carcinoma cells.[5] Adenocarcinoma and malignant melanoma are the most common solid tumors to metastasize to the leptomeninges. Leptomeningeal metastases develop in approximately 5% of patients with breast cancer, 9–25% of cases with small-cell lung cancer and in 23% of patients with melanoma.[5–10]

Patients with acute lymphoblastic leukemia, acute myelogenous leukemia and non-Hodgkin's lymphoma are also at high risk of meningeal involvement. In the early 1970s, as chemotherapy for acute lymphoblastic leukemia became more effective, leukemic meningitis appeared with increasing frequency until almost 50% of the children who had been treated for acute lymphoblastic leukemia developed leptomeningeal metastases. Prophylactic treatment was then instituted to the CNS, and leptomeningeal leukemia became a much less common complication of this illness.[11–13] Leptomeningeal metastases are rarely seen in Hodgkin's disease; however, the most common form of CNS presentation of acquired immune deficiency syndrome-related non-Hodgkin's lymphoma is either asymptomatic or symptomatic lymphomatous leptomeningitis.[14]

Primary brain tumors such as medulloblastoma, ependymoma and germinoma may also metastasize to the meninges. The diffuse or multifocal seeding of the leptomeninges by gliomatous cells is referred to as "meningeal gliomatosis".[15] The leptomeninges become infiltrated by malignant cells from spread of an intracranial malignant glioma by way of the CSF pathways.[15,16]

The means by which systemic tumor reaches the leptomeninges is not entirely clear. Several mechanisms have been proposed. According to one of these mechanisms, the hematogenous spread of tumor cells to the subarachnoid space is via the thin-walled microscopic veins in the arachnoid membranes. Autopsies of patients with leukemic meningitis have demonstrated a predictable pattern of involvement which begins at the walls of superficial arachnoid veins, progresses to the surrounding adventitia and then extends into the CSF. Leukemic cells are also seen deep within the brain in the Virchow–Robin spaces. Experimental models have demonstrated leukemic cell migration through arachnoid vessels.[6,11,17–19] Once malignant cells metastasize to the meninges, they can spread along the surface of the brain and spinal cord and exfoliate tumor cells, which are carried by the flow of spinal fluid throughout the central nervous system. As such, the most frequently affected areas of the CNS are the basilar cisterns, the posterior fossa and the cauda equina where slow CSF flow and gravity promote deposition of circulating tumor cells.[6] Another proposed mechanism for how tumor cells reach the leptomeninges is by hematogenous metastases to the choroid plexus with subsequent rupture into the CSF.[19] In the presence of brain parenchymal metastases, meningeal malignant infiltration may result as a direct extension from an underlying parenchymal lesion. In the case of metastatic lesions in the skull or vertebral bodies, tumor cells may spread via the perivascular spaces of the intravertebral veins or the venous plexus and subsequently along the radicular veins to the subarachnoid space.[20] In autopsy studies of patients with small-cell lung cancer, leptomeningeal metastases were often focal and adjacent to the involved brain or spinal cord suggesting secondary invasion of the leptomeninges from the primary metastases.[21] The choroid plexus is frequently involved when small-cell lung cancer metastasizes to the CNS. Tumor cells may enter the subarachnoid space at the spinal level along nerve roots. In autopsy studies of patients with small-cell lung cancer with isolated leptomeningeal disease, involvement of perineural and perivascular lymphatics, and invasion of endoneural and perineural sheaths of the intervertebral foramina have been demonstrated.[6,8,21] Ependymomas, pineoblastomas and medulloblastomas, which are in continuity with the CSF, frequently metastasize to the meninges via the CSF. Similarly, parenchymal brain tumors that are in continuity with the cerebral ventricles can rupture into the CSF.

Tumor which has seeded the leptomeninges either grows in a linear pattern, creating a thin layer of cells that is spread diffusely over the surface of the brain and spinal cord, or meningeal tumor may assume a nodular growth pattern, with areas of subarachnoid tumor nodules and intervening tumor-free areas. Collections of tumor cells in the leptomeninges that are more than a few cells thick establish their own capillary supply (neovascularization) which does not have a blood–brain barrier. For this reason, leptomeningeal metastases are readily demonstrated by contrast-enhanced computed tomography scan or gadolinium-enhanced magnetic resonance imaging. This also has implications for treatment as systemic chemotherapy should be able to reach these tumor cells via the tumor's own blood supply.[11]

References

1. Eberth CJ. Zur Entwicklung des Epithelioms (Cholesteatoms) der Pia und der Lunge. *Virchows Arch* 1870; **49:** 51–62.
2. Oppenheim H. Uber Hirnsymptome bei Carcinomatose ohne nachweisbare Veranderungen in Gehirn. *Charite-Annalen* 1888; **13:** 335–44.
3. Siefert E. Uber die multiple Karzinomatose des Zentralnervensystems. *Munch Med Wochenschr* 1902; **49:** 826–8.
4. Beerman WF. Meningeal carcinomatosis. *JAMA* 1912; **58:** 1437–9.
5. Little JR, Dale AJD, Okazaki H. Meningeal carcinomatosis: clinical manifestations. *Arch Neurol* 1974; **30:** 138–43.
6. Grossman SA, Moynihan TJ. Neoplastic meningitis. *Neurol Clin* 1991; **9:** 843–56.
7. Amer MH, Al Sarraf M, Baker LH, et al. Malignant melanoma and central nervous system metastases. *Cancer* 1978; **42:** 660–8.
8. Aroney RS, Dalley DN, Chan WK, et al. Meningeal carcinomatosis in small cell carcinoma of the lung. *Am J Med* 1981; **71:** 26–32.
9. Grant R, Naylor B, Greenberg HS, Junck L. Clinical outcome in aggressively treated meningeal carcinomatosis. *Arch Neurol* 1994; **51:** 457–61.
10. Theodore WH, Gendelman S. Meningeal carcinomatosis. *Arch Neurol* 1981; **38:** 696–9.
11. Wasserstrom WR, Glass JP, Posner JB. Diagnosis and treatment of leptomeningeal metastases from solid tumors: experience with 90 patients. *Cancer* 1982; **49:** 759–72.
12. Nies BA, Thomas LB, Freireich EJ. Meningeal leukemia: a follow-up study. *Cancer* 1965; **18:** 546–53.
13. Simone J. Acute lymphocytic leukemia in childhood. *Sem Hematol* 1974; **11:** 25–39.
14. Berger JR, Levy RM. The neurologic complications of human immunodeficiency virus isolation. *Med Clin North Amer* 1993; **77:** 1–23.
15. Yung WA, Horten BC, Shapiro WR. Meningeal gliomatosis: a review of 12 cases. *Ann Neurol* 1980; **8:** 605–8.
16. Ho KL, Hoschner JA, Wolfe DE. Primary leptomeningeal gliomatosis: symptoms suggestive of meningitis. *Arch Neurol* 1981; **38:** 662–6.
17. Price RA, Johnson WW. The central nervous system in childhood leukemia. I. The arachnoid. *Cancer* 1973; **31:** 520–33.
18. Azzarelli B, Mirkin LD, Goheen M. The leptomeningeal vein-A site of re-entry of leukemic cells into the systemic circulation. *Cancer* 1984; **54:** 1333–43.
19. Grain GO, Karr JP. Diffuse leptomeningeal carcinomatosis: clinical and pathologic characteristics. *Neurology* 1955; **5:** 706–22.
20. Boogerd W, Hart AAM, van der Sande JJ, Engelsman E. Meningeal carcinomatosis in breast cancer: prognostic factors and influence of treatment. *Cancer* 1991; **67:** 1685–95.
21. Rosen ST, Aisner J, Makuch RW, et al. Carcinomatous leptomeningitis in small cell lung cancer: a clinicopathologic review of the National Cancer Institute experience. *Medicine* (Baltimore) 1982; **61:** 45–53.

96.   *Leptomeningeal metastases are manifest clinically by headache, encephalopathy, cranial neuropathies and radiculopathies*

The clinical presentation of leptomeningeal metastases depends on the extent of disease along the neuraxis. Wasserstrom et al.[1] describe the clinical signs and symptoms of leptomeningeal metastases in 90 patients by symptoms and signs referrable to brain involvement, cranial nerve involvement and spinal cord or spinal nerve root involvement (Tables 96.1 and 96.2).[1-3] In most series, headache is the most frequent complaint. It is typically described as severe, constant, either diffuse or located at the base of the skull with radiation into the neck, and frequently is worse when the patient awakens in the morning. There is often associated neck pain and stiffness, though the meningismus is much less severe than that described in purulent meningitis. Headache is often associated with nausea and vomiting, and light-headedness. Cognitive abnormalities consisting of lethargy, confusion or memory loss are also common initial complaints. Focal or generalized seizures may develop.

Table 96.1   Leptomeningeal metastases: symptoms

	Wasserstrom et al. ($n = 90$)	Theodore et al. ($n = 33$)	Aroney et al. ($n = 11$)
Brain			
Headache	30	13	2
Lethargy, confusion, memory loss	15	18	8
Nausea/vomiting	10	4	
Cranial nerves			
Diplopia	18		
Hearing loss	7		
Spinal nerves			
Backache	23	8	7
Radicular pain	19		
Difficulty walking	12		
Paresthesias	31		
Bowel/bladder dysfunction	12		5

The symptom of headache may be due to hydrocephalus with increased intracranial pressure. Tumor that settles in the basilar cisterns often interferes with the flow of CSF from the ventricular system to the cerebral convexities with resultant obstructive and/or communicating hydrocephalus.

Table 96.2   Leptomeningeal metastases: signs

	Wasserstrom et al. (n = 90)	Theodore et al. (n = 33)	Aroney et al. (n = 11)
Nuchal rigidity	7	11	
Cognitive abnormalities	28		5
Seizures	5	1	
Cranial-nerve abnormalities			
Ocular muscle paresis (III, IV, VI)	18	13	
Facial weakness (VII)	15	10	
Decreased hearing (VIII)	9	1	
Papilledema	5	7	
Dysphagia, hoarseness, diminished gag	8	10	
Spinal-nerve root abnormalities			
Extremity weakness	54	18	2
Reflex asymmetry	64	8	
Sensory loss	24	11	4
Decreased rectal tone	10		

In one review of 33 cases of meningeal carcinomatosis, cranial nerve abnormalities accounted for 79% of the findings on neurologic examination. These included ocular motility abnormalities, nystagmus, facial paresis and sensory loss, dysarthria, dysphagia and hoarseness.[2] In Wasserstrom's series,[1] cranial nerve abnormalities were present in 35 of 90 patients (39%) at initial evaluation. The most common complaints were diplopia, hearing loss, facial numbness and loss of visual acuity. On examination there was evidence of cranial nerve abnormalities in 50 (56%) of the patients, the most frequent being ocular muscle paresis. In a review of the clinical symptomatology in 29 cases of meningeal carcinomatosis, cranial nerve involvement was present in 21 patients.[4]

In all series, signs of spinal nerve root involvement is one of the most frequent abnormalities on initial examination. The most common complaints are either weakness, usually affecting the legs, pain in the back or neck with or without radicular pain, and paresthesias in one or more extremities. In Wasserstrom's series,[1] approximately 70% of patients had signs of spinal nerve root involvement on initial examination characterized primarily by asymmetries of deep tendon reflexes (64 patients) or evidence of a cauda equina syndrome (30 patients). In Little's series[4] of 29 cases of meningeal carcinomatosis, 94% of patients had signs of spinal nerve root involvement. The most common signs were lower extremity weakness and atrophy with sensory deficits and areflexia. Spinal nerve root involvement affecting the lower extremities is much more common than spinal nerve root involvement of the upper extremities. This is related, in part, to the gravitation of malignant cells in the CSF into the cul-de-sac of the thecal sac, the slow flow of CSF in this region and the fact that the nerve roots comprising the cauda equina have an extensive course in the subarachnoid space.[4] Similarly, in Theodore's series,[2] signs of spinal nerve root involvement were present in 18 of 33 patients with meningeal carcinomatosis. The symptoms and signs of leptomeningeal metastases are listed in Tables 96.1 and 96.2.

In all series, the interval from the diagnosis of the primary malignancy (carcinoma of the breast, lung or malignant melanoma) to the diagnosis of leptomeningeal metastases varies considerably. In general, the diagnosis of leptomeningeal involvement is made 6 months to 3 years after the discovery of the primary tumor. In some patients, however, the diagnosis of the primary tumor is made at the time of the presentation of leptomeningeal metastases with neurologic symptoms and signs, while in other patients the diagnosis of leptomeningeal metastases is made 10 years or more after the primary tumor was discovered.[1,2]

References

1. Wasserstrom WR, Glass JP, Posner JB. Diagnosis and treatment of leptomeningeal metastases from solid tumors: experience with 90 patients. *Cancer* 1982; **49:** 759–72.
2. Theodore WH, Gendelman S. Meningeal carcinomatosis. *Arch Neurol* 1981; **38:** 696–9.
3. Aroney RS, Dalley DN, Chan WK, Bell DR, Levi JA. Meningeal carcinomatosis in small cell carcinoma of the lung. *Amer J Med* 1981; **71:** 26–32.
4. Little JR, Dale AJD, Okazaki H. Meningeal carcinomatosis: clinical manifestations. *Arch Neurol* 1974; **30:** 138–43.

97.   *Examination of the CSF is the single most important test for the diagnosis of leptomeningeal metastases*

The presence of leptomeningeal metastases is suspected by the clinical presentation, supported by evidence of meningeal enhancement post-contrast administration on computed tomography (CT) or magnetic resonance imaging (MRI), and established by the identification of malignant cells in the CSF.

On examination of the CSF, the opening pressure is typically elevated, the protein concentration is moderately to markedly increased and the glucose concentration is either normal or low. The protein concentration may be very high in the CSF; values in the range of 2,000–3,000 mg/dL are not unheard of. A nonspecific pleocytosis, consisting of lymphocytes, monocytes and polymorphonuclear leukocytes, is presumably a reaction to the tumor in the leptomeninges. Malignant cells will be identified in the CSF on initial lumbar puncture in approximately 50–70% of patients (Table 97.1).[1-3] A second lumbar puncture increases the yield of positive CSF cytology to 80–90%.[1-3] The optimum amount of CSF for cytology is 10 mL or greater. In general, the incidence of positive CSF cytology is higher in CSF obtained from a lumbar puncture than from a cisternal puncture. However, on occasion, cisternal CSF may be positive when lumbar CSF is negative. A false-negative CSF cytology may be due to inadequate volume, inefficient handling or poor site selection. Obtain CSF from a site along the neuraxis close to the area of symptomatic disease. In the presence of encephalopathy or cranial neuropathies, CSF should be obtained from a cisternal puncture. In the presence of a cauda equina syndrome, CSF should be sampled from a lumbar interspace.

Table 97.1   Cerebrospinal fluid abnormalities in meningeal carcinomatosis

	Little et al. (n=21)	Theodore et al.* (n=33)	Wasserstrom et al.** (n=90)
Cerebrospinal fluid pressure >180 mmH$_2$O		10	45
Protein >45 mg/dL	12	24	73
Glucose <45 mg/dL	16	18	28
WBCs >5/mm^3	10	19	51
Positive cytology	17	24	49
Normal			3

*Cerebrospinal fluid cell counts ranged from 0 to 550 cells/mm^3, protein concentrations from 33 mg/dL to 2.3 g/dL.
**Cerebrospinal fluid cell counts ranged from 0 to 1800 cells/mm^3, protein concentrations ranged from 24 to 2485 mg/dL.

Malignant cells in the CSF produce biochemical substances. The identification of these biochemical tumor markers in CSF is helpful in the diagnosis of leptomeningeal metastases in the absence of a positive cytology. A CSF beta-glucuronidase concentration > 80 mU/L is strongly suggestive of the presence of leptomeningeal metastases.[3,4] Elevations in the CSF concentration of beta-glucuronidase are also seen in acute and chronic infectious meningitis.[5-7] In Wasserstrom's series,[3] CSF beta-glucuronidase levels above 80 mU/L were found in 13 of 17 patients with leptomeningeal metastases from carcinoma of the breast, 6 of 9 patients with carcinoma of the lung and 2 of 4 patients with malignant melanoma.

Carcinoembryonic antigen (CEA) is a high molecular weight glycoprotein produced by colon, breast, ovarian, bladder and lung cancer cells. An elevated

CSF CEA above 1 ng/mL without a concomitant elevated serum CEA level above 100 ng/mL is relatively specific for carcinomatous meningitis. This marker can also be used to monitor response to therapy as it tends to decline with successful therapy.[5,8–10] The CSF lactate concentration may be elevated; however, as has been discussed (see maxim 24), an elevated CSF lactate concentration is a nonspecific abnormality and occurs in bacterial meningitis, stroke, head injury, primary CNS tumors, following seizure activity, in subarachnoid hemorrhage, and in tuberculous meningitis.

The diagnosis of leptomeningeal metastases can be made, on occasion, based on clinical criteria alone in patients with a known cancer, and signs and symptoms of neurologic dysfunction at multiple levels of the neuraxis. The vast majority of patients, however, have either laboratory evidence or neuroimaging evidence of leptomeningeal involvement. The appearance of diffuse meningeal enhancement following contrast administration on either a CT scan or MRI (Fig. 97.1), with or without hydrocephalus, or the

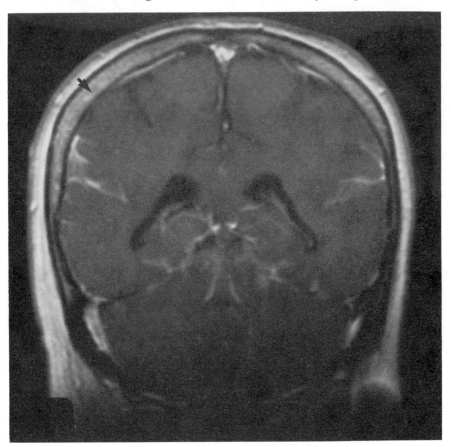

Fig. 97.1   Carcinomatous meningitis. T_1-weighted cranial magnetic resonance scan post-gadolinium administration demonstrating diffuse meningeal enhancement (black arrow).

appearance of multiple enhancing subarachnoid nodules (Fig. 97.2) in a patient with a known cancer is highly suggestive of the diagnosis of leptomeningeal metastases. The gadolinium-enhanced MRI is the most sensitive technique for identifying leptomeningeal enhancement.

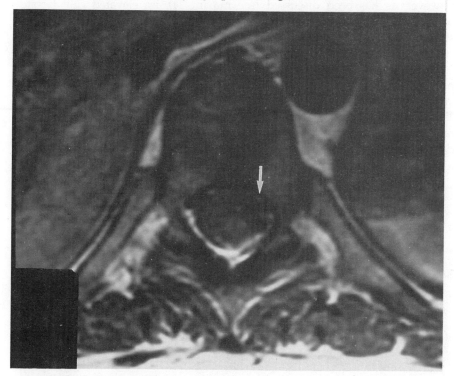

Fig. 97.2 Carcinomatous meningitis. T_1-weighted spinal magnetic resonance scan post-gadolinium demonstrating multiple enhancing subarachnoid nodules (white arrow).

References

1. Little JR, Dale AJD, Okazaki H. Meningeal carcinomatosis. *Arch Neurol* 1974; **30:** 138–43.
2. Theodore WH, Gendelman S. Meningeal carcinomatosis. *Arch Neurol* 1981; **38:** 696–9.
3. Wasserstrom WR, Glass JP, Posner JB. Diagnosis and treatment of leptomeningeal metastases from solid tumors: experience with 90 patients. *Cancer* 1982; **49:** 759–72.
4. Schold SC, Wasserstrom WR, Fleisher M, Schwartz M, Posner JB. Cerebrospinal fluid biochemical markers of central nervous system metastases. *Ann Neurol* 1980; **8:** 597–604.
5. Grossman SA, Moynihan TJ. Neoplastic meningitis. *Neurol Clin* 1991; **9:** 843–56.
6. Shuttleworth E, Allen N. CSF beta-glucuronidase assay in the diagnosis of neoplastic meningitis. *Arch Neurol* 1980; **37:** 684–7.
7. Tallman RD, Kimbrough SM, OBrien JF, et al. Assay for beta-glucuronidase in

cerebrospinal fluid: usefulness for the detection of neoplastic meningitis. *Mayo Clin Proc* 1985; **60:** 293–8.

8. Jacobi C, Reiber H, Felgenhauer K. The clinical relevance of locally produced carcinoembryonic antigen in cerebrospinal fluid. *J Neurol* 1986; **233:** 358–61.

9. Klee GG, Tallman RD, Goellner JR, et al. Elevation of carcinoembryonic antigen in cerebrospinal fluid among patients with meningeal carcinomatosis. *Mayo Clin Proc* 1986; **61:** 9–13.

10. Yap BS, Yap HY, Fritsche HA, et al. CSF carcinoembryonic antigen in meningeal carcinomatosis from breast cancer. *JAMA* 1980; **244:** 1601–3.

98.   *The standard therapy for leptomeningeal metastases from solid tumors is radiotherapy to symptomatic areas and intrathecal chemotherapy*

The median survival from the time of diagnosis of leptomeningeal metastases is 4–6 weeks, unless aggressive treatment is initiated.[1,2] The purpose of treatment is to prolong survival and to stabilize neurologic function. The standard therapy for carcinomatous meningitis is radiotherapy to symptomatic areas followed by intrathecal chemotherapy. Radiation therapy (RT) of the entire neuraxis may produce severe marrow suppression preventing the subsequent use of chemotherapeutic agents. In addition, while acute leukemia is a highly radiosensitive tumor and whole-neuraxis radiation therapy is a very effective treatment, adenocarcinoma of the breast and lung is a less radiosensitive tumor. For these reasons it is recommended that focal radiation therapy be given to the areas of most symptomatic disease, and to the regions in which neuroimaging studies have demonstrated bulk disease or where a radionuclide CSF flow study has demonstrated areas of obstruction to the flow of CSF.

It is preferable to administer intrathecal chemotherapy through a subcutaneous reservoir with a ventricular catheter. The most common subcutaneous reservoir in use today is the Ommaya reservoir. The subcutaneous reservoir is connected to the frontal horn of the lateral ventricle by a catheter (Fig. 98.1). The advantages of using the Ommaya reservoir over repeated lumbar punctures are:

1. Intraventricular injection of the chemotherapeutic agent via the reservoir assures that the material enters the CSF. Chemotherapeutic agents injected via lumbar puncture may be inadvertently injected into the subdural or epidural space.
2. Chemotherapeutic agents injected into the ventricle follow the normal pathways of CSF flow (provided the flow of CSF is normal). Shapiro et al.[3] demonstrated that methotrexate injected into the lumbar sac did not reach the ventricular areas in therapeutic concentrations.
3. In the treatment of acute leptomeningeal leukemia, two studies which compared the efficacy of methotrexate given by lumbar puncture with

methotrexate given by ventricular instillation demonstrated that the drug given by an Ommaya device produced a longer remission of the leptomeningeal disease.[4,5]

4. Repetitive lumbar punctures are unpleasant for the patient.[2,3]

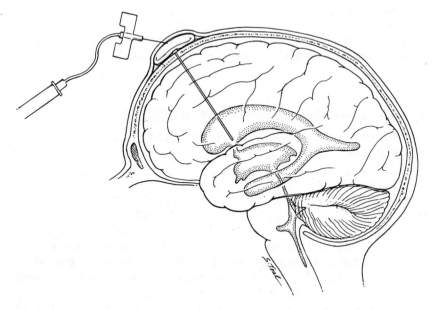

Fig. 98.1 Ommaya reservoir for the administration of intrathecal chemotherapy.

There are three chemotherapeutic agents used for intrathecal chemotherapy: methotrexate, cytosine arabinoside and thiotepa. Methotrexate is the most frequently used chemotherapeutic agent used in most protocols because cytosine arabinoside is not effective against most solid tumors (although it is extensively used in leukemic and lymphomatous meningitis), and thiotepa is rapidly eliminated from the CSF. Methotrexate levels can be measured in CSF, and most treatment protocols are based on frequent sampling of CSF from the Ommaya device, injecting methotrexate when the CSF concentration has fallen below a "therapeutic level".[6] Ongerboer de Visser et al.[6] reported neurologic improvement in 80% of 19 breast cancer patients treated with intraventricular methotrexate therapy with a median survival of 6 months (25% of the patients survived 1 year or more). In their treatment protocol, 5 mg of methotrexate was injected whenever ventricular CSF levels fell below 1×10^3 nmol/L, until no tumor cells were seen in the ventricular samples. Cerebrospinal fluid samples were withdrawn daily from an Ommaya device for methotrexate determination. When tumor cells were no longer present, methotrexate 5 mg was given three additional times, and then the treatment interval was increased to 4–6 weeks, and finally to 4–6 months. Wasserstrom et al.[2] reported neurologic improvement or neurologic stabilization in 28 of 46 breast cancer patients (61%) that lasted from 2 to 20 months. The median survival was 7 months. The treatment protocol consisted of radiation therapy using 2,400 rads in eight doses over 10–14 days directed to the site of major clinical involvement. Prior to, or immediately after, the completion of RT, an Ommaya reservoir was placed. Methotrexate (7 mg/m^2 body surface) was instilled twice a week for five treatments. Citrovorum factor (9 mg)was given orally every 12 hours on the day of treatment and 3 days following treatment. Intraventricular instillation was performed twice weekly until there was evidence of cytologic improvement or clinical stabilization. At that time chemotherapy was given once weekly on an outpatient basis. If improvement continued, the treatment interval was lengthened to every 2, 3 or 4 weeks.[2]

There appears to be no clearcut benefit to using more than one intrathecal chemotherapeutic agent. Giannone et al.[7] investigated a biweekly combination of intraventricular chemotherapy using methotrexate, cytosine arabinoside and thiotepa in patients with meningeal metastases from breast cancer, lung cancer, non-Hodgkin's lymphoma, malignant melanoma and bladder carcinoma. The primary goal was to evaluate the toxicity of this regimen. The dose of each drug was comparable to that studied as a single agent in the treatment of meningeal metastases and lymphoma. The major adverse effect was myelosuppression, which occurred in 17 of 22 patients (77%); in 13 of these patients the myelosuppression was life-threatening, and developed during the 4 weeks of treatment. The triple-drug intraventricular chemotherapy did not increase the response rate or survival when compared with single agent methotrexate and radiotherapy.[7]

Carcinoma of the lung that metastasizes to the meninges includes many histologic types such as small-cell carcinoma, adenocarcinoma, squamous-cell carcinoma and poorly differentiated large-cell carcinoma. Patients with leptomeningeal metastases from lung carcinomas can be treated as described above with a combination of radiation therapy and intraventricular methotrexate.

Central nervous system metastases from non-Hodgkin's lymphoma is usually followed by systemic relapse within a few months. Therefore, patients with apparently isolated CNS relapse should be considered to have systemic relapse as well and should receive systemic therapy in addition to conventional CNS treatment. Survival in patients with CNS lymphoma is related to systemic and not to CNS disease. Radiotherapy has been a mainstay of treatment. Radiation therapy may, however, be withheld in asymptomatic patients where there is no evidence of heavy local infiltration of tumor in the meninges by clinical or radiographic examination. Methotrexate is the recommended chemotherapy via an Ommaya reservoir. In patients who develop toxicity to methotrexate, cytosine arabinoside may be substituted.[8,9]

A standard treatment protocol for leptomeningeal metastases from solid tumors requires methotrexate to be given in a dose of 10–12 mg, initially twice a week for 4–6 weeks, or until CSF cytology is negative, followed by weekly and then monthly maintenance therapy. Oral leucovorin is routinely given following each methotrexate injection.[10] A cumulative dose of 150 mg methotrexate should not be exceeded.[11]

Increasing interest is developing in treating leptomeningeal metastases with systemic chemotherapy. As has been discussed, these deposits are highly vascularized tumors and, therefore, systemic therapy would obtain access to the subarachnoid mass through its own blood supply.[12] Siegal et al.[10] demonstrated the effectiveness of systemic chemotherapy alone in 7 patients with leptomeningeal metastases from solid tumors. The median survival of 14 breast cancer patients treated with systemic chemotherapy, radiation therapy and hormonal therapy was as long as the median survival of 44 breast cancer patients treated with intraventricular chemotherapy (12 weeks). Six patients (43%) survived 6 months or more and 2 patients survived for longer than 1 year.[1]

References

1. Boogerd W, Hart AAM, van der Sande JJ, Engelsman E. Meningeal carcinomatosis in breast cancer: prognostic factors and influence of treatment. *Cancer* 1991; **67**: 1685–95.
2. Wasserstrom WR, Glass JP, Posner JB. Diagnosis and treatment of leptomeningeal metastases from solid tumors: experience with 90 patients. *Cancer* 1982; **49**: 759–72.
3. Shapiro WR, Young DF, Mehta BP. Methotrexate distribution in cerebrospinal fluid after intravenous, ventricular and lumbar injections. *N Engl J Med* 1975; **293**: 161–6.
4. Bleyer WA, Poplack DG. Intraventricular versus intralumbar methotrexate for central-nervous-system leukemia: prolonged remission with the Ommaya reservoir. *Med Ped Oncol* 1979; **6**: 207–13.
5. Shapiro WR, Posner JB, Ushio Y, et al. Treatment of meningeal neoplasms. *Cancer Treat Rep* 1977; **61**: 733–43.
6. Ongerboer de Visser BW, Somers R, Nooyen WH, Van Heerde P, Hart AAM, McVie G. Intraventricular methotrexate therapy of the leptomeningeal metastasis from breast carcinoma. *Neurology* 1983; **33**: 1365–72.
7. Giannone L, Greco FA, Hainsworth JD. Combination intraventricular chemotherapy for meningeal neoplasia. *J Clin Oncol* 1986; **4**: 68–73.
8. Recht L, Straus DJ, Cirrincione C, Thaler HT, Posner JB. Central nervous system metastases from non-Hodgkin's lymphoma: treatment and prophylaxis. *Am J Med* 1988; **84**: 425–35.
9. Macintosh F, Colby T, Podolsky W, et al. Central nervous system involvement in non-Hodgkin's lymphoma: an analysis of 105 cases. *Cancer* 1982; **49**: 586–95.
10. Siegal T, Lossos A, Pfeffer MR. Leptomeningeal metastases: analysis of 31 patients with sustained off-therapy response following combined-modality therapy. *Neurology* 1994; **44**: 1463–9.
11. Storch-Hagenlocher B, Herrmann R, Schabet M. Carcinomatous and leukemic meningitis. In: Hacke W (ed.), *NeuroCritical Care*. Berlin: Springer-Verlag, 1994; 743–8.
12. Siegal T, Sandbank U, Gabizon A, et al. Alteration of blood–brain–CSF barrier in experimental meningeal carcinomatosis: a morphologic and adriamycin-penetration study. *J Neurooncol* 1987; **4**: 233–42.

99.   *The most common complications of intrathecal chemotherapy are infection and leukoencephalopathy*

The complications of the use of intrathecal chemotherapy can be divided into complications of intraventricular reservoirs and the neurotoxicity of intrathecal chemotherapy.

Obbens et al.[1] reviewed the records of 387 patients with cancer who had Ommaya reservoirs. Infection was one of the main complications, and was usually caused by *Staphylococcus aureus* and coagulase-negative staphylococci. Most of these infections were treated successfully with intravenous or intraventricular antibiotics, or both, without removing the reservoir. Pericatheter necrosis developed in two patients after repeated intraventricular chemotherapy. In both cases a necrotic mass was detected around the catheter tract and was thought to be due to leakage of drugs into the cerebral white matter around the catheter tract.[1] In a review of 61 cases of intraventricular reservoir use for intrathecal chemotherapy, infectious complications developed in 14 (23%). Twelve patients had meningitis and 2 patients had a local cellulitis at the site of the intraventricular reservoir. *Propionibacterium acnes* and staphylococci were responsible for 75% of the cases of meningitis.[2]

The neurotoxicity of intrathecal methotrexate is well known. In one series, leukoencephalopathy developed in 16 of 27 patients (59%) treated with intrathecal methotrexate. The diagnosis was based on a computed tomography (CT) scan appearance of hypodensity either surrounding the indwelling catheter or of the periventricular white matter. Symptoms and signs of leukoencephalopathy included apathy, abnormalities of cognitive function, motor and gait dysfunction, and seizures. When the group of patients with leukoencephalopathy was compared with the group of patients who were treated with intrathecal chemotherapy but did not develop leukoencephalopathy, the groups differed in only one aspect. An elevated opening CSF pressure was measured at diagnosis in 50% of the patients in the leukoencephalopathy group, whereas in the patients without leukoencephalopathy, only 18% had an initial elevated opening pressure ($P<0.05$).[3] The increased intracranial pressure was attributed to ventricular outlet obstruction and abnormal CSF flow which most likely affected the distribution of the methotrexate. In Boogerd's series[4] of breast cancer patients with meningeal carcinomatosis, leukoencephalopathy developed in 11 of the 17 patients who survived more than 4 months. In 9 of these 11 patients, leukoencephalopathy sooner or later progressed to a serious disability that became a major contributing factor to death.

The leukoencephalopathy associated with intrathecal methotrexate is characterized by demyelination of the deep white matter in the periventricular regions and centrum semiovale with sparing of the grey matter and basal ganglia.[5] The combination of cranial irradiation, systemic and intrathecal methotrexate significantly increases the risk of leukoencephalopathy.[6]

The risk of leukoencephalopathy from the combination of radiation therapy and intrathecal methotrexate is greatest when radiation therapy is given immediately before, or simultaneously with, intrathecal methotrexate.[7,8] The most frequent signs and symptoms of methotrexate leukoencephalopathy are confusion, drooling, stupor or irritability, ataxia, tremors, seizures, spasticity and slurred speech. The CT scan will demonstrate low-density nonenhancing areas in the periventricular white matter.[8] Examination of CSF from children with leukoencephalopathy demonstrated an elevated concentration of myelin basic protein, suggesting active demyelination.[8,9]

Patients may also experience symptoms of "meningeal irritation" associated with the intraventricular administration of methotrexate. Symptoms of stiff neck, headache, nausea and vomiting, fever and lethargy begin 2–4 hours after injection and last for 12–72 hours.[8]

Boogerd et al.[4] reported symptoms of headache, nausea, dizziness and fever in 10 of 44 patients in the first weeks of intraventricular methotrexate treatment. Examination of the CSF was normal and cultures were negative. Others have observed a CSF pleocytosis with this syndrome.[10,11] A "somnolence syndrome" is also described consisting of the rapid onset of lethargy, low-grade fever, nausea and vomiting, and accompanied by generalized slowing of the background activity on electroencephalogram. This syndrome typically begins 3–8 weeks after completion of CNS prophylaxis with cranial irradiation and intrathecal methotrexate. It is typically observed in patients who have received both radiation and intrathecal therapy, but has also been reported in patients receiving cranial irradiation only. The syndrome usually resolves within 1 to 4 weeks.[8,12,13]

References

1. Obbens E, Leavens ME, Beal JW, Lee YY. Ommaya reservoirs in 387 cancer patients: a 15-year experience. *Neurology* 1985; **35:** 1274–8.
2. Browne MJ, Dinndorf PA, Perek D, Commers J, et al. Infectious complications of intraventricular reservoirs in cancer patients. *Pediatr Infect Dis J* 1987; **6:** 182–9.
3. Siegal T, Lossos A, Pfeffer MR. Leptomeningeal metastases: analysis of 31 patients with sustained off-therapy response following combined-modality therapy. *Neurology* 1994; **44:** 1463–9.
4. Boogerd W, Hart AAM, van der Sande JJ, Engelsman E. Meningeal carcinomatosis in breast cancer: prognostic factors and influence of treatment. *Cancer* 1991; **67:** 1685–95.
5. Liu HM, Maurer HS, Vongsvivut S, Conway JJ. Methotrexate encephalopathy, a neuropathologic study. *Hum Pathol* 1978; **9:** 635–48.
6. McIntosh S, Rothman S, Rosenfield N, et al. Systemic methotrexate and chronic neurotoxicity in childhood leukemia – a preliminary report. *Proc Am Assoc Cancer Res* 1978; **19:** 362.
7. Price RA, Jamieson PA. The central nervous system in childhood leukemia II. Subacute leucoencephalopathy. *Cancer* 1975; **35:** 306–18.
8. Kaplan RS, Wiernik PH. Neurotoxicity of antineoplastic drugs. *Semin Oncol* 1982; **9:** 103–30.
9. Gangji D, Reaman GH, Cohen SR, et al. Leukoencephalopathy and elevated levels of myelin basic protein in the cerebrospinal fluid of patients with acute lymphoblastic leukemia. *N Engl J Med* 1980; **303:** 19–21.

10. Mott MG, Stevenson P, Wood CBC. Methotrexate meningitis. *Lancet* 1972; **2**: 656.
11. Geiser CF, Bishop Y, Jaffe N, et al. Adverse effects of intrathecal methotrexate in children with acute leukemia in remission. *Blood* 1975; **45**: 180–95.
12. Parker D, Malpas JS, Sandland R, et al. Sequelae of central nervous system prophylaxis. In Whitehouse JMA, Kay HEM (eds), *CNS Complications of Malignant Disease*. Baltimore: University Park, 1979; 227–35.
13. Inati A, Sallan S, Cassady JR, et al. Effects of central nervous system prophylaxis in childhood acute lymphoblastic leukemia. *Proc Am Assoc Cancer Res and ASCO* 1981; **22**: 388.

100.   *Gliomas that arise in the leptomeninges, so-called primary leptomeningeal gliomatosis, are rare*

The bulk of this chapter has been dedicated to leptomeningeal metastases from solid tumors. Gliomas arising primarily in the leptomeninges are rare with less than 20 cases reported in the literature.[1-5] Primary leptomeningeal gliomas are due to neoplastic transformation of the cellular elements of heterotopic glial nests in the subarachnoid space.[6] Heterotopic leptomeningeal neuroglial tissue is composed primarily of astrocytes, neuroglial fibers, oligodendrocytes and small ependyma-lined canals.[1,2,7] Although the leptomeninges are diffusely infiltrated by neoplastic cells, this pathologic process is entirely confined to the subarachnoid space with no extension into the brain or spinal cord parenchyma. The symptoms of primary leptomeningeal gliomatosis are due to increased intracranial pressure as the flow of CSF is interrupted by subarachnoid macroscopic deposits (nests of astrocytes and glial fibers) and thickening of the meninges with resultant obstructive hydrocephalus. Characteristic symptoms are headache, blurred vision, nausea and vomiting, seizures and an altered level of consciousness. Lethargy, confusion, papilledema and cranial nerve abnormalities are common. Examination of the CSF demonstrates an elevated opening pressure, a marked elevation in the protein concentration with values of 900–1000 mg/dL reported, a lymphocytic pleocytosis and a low glucose concentration. Neuroimaging may demonstrate dilatation of the ventricular system with nodular or diffuse enhancement of the meninges. In the majority of the reported cases of primary leptomeningeal gliomatosis, cytologic examination of the CSF was negative and the diagnosis was made based on histologic examination at autopsy.[1,5,6]

The rarity of this condition and the difficulty in making the diagnosis mean that the role of chemotherapy and radiation therapy is not known. The cause of death is obstructive hydrocephalus with raised intracranial pressure and brainstem compression. Ventriculoperitoneal shunting may be beneficial as a temporary measure but, as the meningeal process progresses and the flow of CSF is obstructed at the foramina of Monro and the cerebral aqueduct, shunting is of little benefit.

References

1. Ho KL, Hoschner JA, Wolfe DE. Primary leptomeningeal gliomatosis. *Arch Neurol* 1981; **38:** 662–6.
2. Cooper IS, Craig WM, Kernohan JW. Tumors of the spinal cord: primary extramedullary gliomas. *Surg Gynecol Obstet* 1951; **92:** 183–90.
3. Daum S, Le Beau J, Billet R. Sus-tentorial gliomas: an extra-cerebral development. *Neurochirurgie* 1963; **9:** 279–88.
4. Abbott KH, Glass B. Intracranial extracerebral (leptomeningeal) glioma: report of case and review of literature. *Proceedings of the Second International Congress on Neuropathology: Part I.* Amsterdam: Excerpta Medica, 1955; 165–8.
5. Scully RE, Galdabini JJ, McNeely BU. Case 44, Case Records of the Massachusetts General Hospital: weekly clinicopathologic exercises. *N Engl J Med* 1978; **299:** 1060–7.
6. Cooper IS, Kernohan JW. Heterotopic glial nests in the subarachnoid space: histopathologic characteristics, mode of origin and relation to meningeal gliomas. *J Neuropathol Exp Neurol* 1951; **10:** 16–29.
7. Popoff N, Feigin I. Heterotopic central nervous tissue in subarachnoid space. *Arch Pathol* 1964; **78:** 533–9.

Index